CHAOS TO CALM

BY
HELEN MELROSE

First published in 2024 by Helen Melrose

Author: Melrose, Helen
Title: Chaos to Calm: Finding Serenity in Turbulent Times

ISBN: 9798884167957

Editor-in-chief: Anita Saunders
Cover Design: Sarah Rose Graphic Design

Disclaimer:
The material in this publication is of the nature of general professional advice, but it is not intended to provide specific guidance for particular circumstances and it should not be relied on as the basis for any decision to take action or not take action on any particular matter which it covers. Readers should obtain individual advice from the author where appropriate, before making any such decision. To the maximum extent permitted by law, the author and publisher disclaim all responsibility and liability to any person, arising directly or indirectly from any person taking or not taking action based on the information in this publication.

DEDICATION

I dedicate this book to the Mother in me and in you. May her qualities of Kindness, Caring, Nurturing, and Strength come to the fore and take the helm of the ship, so as to Gently and Lovingly guide us through the Chaos into a world of Calm.

TABLE OF CONTENTS

FOREWORD

It gave me great pleasure and delight to read Helen Melrose's latest transparent contribution from her own personal experiences, *Chaos to Calm*.

Helen is a very wise and dedicated teacher and seeker of truth, and lives her life as an example by living a peaceful and harmonious existence whilst assisting others to find direction in their Journey of Life.

In a world of confusion, suffering, and destruction Helen reminds us that were we to change the paradigm of our present consciousness, a shift will occur on our precious Earth simultaneously. Unity is the treasure we seek.

Following Helen's example of insights and guidance of cleverly woven words you may well discover that you are here to develop an intimate and magical relationship with yourself, along with others with whom we share this Universe.

Helen, my dear sister of the light, may your honest words and heartfelt story inspire others along the path to Enlightenment.

Marilyn Hannon—Healer, Author *Revelations: The Way It Is*

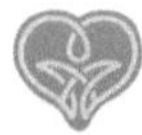

PREFACE

October 16, 2023

Today is a special day for me. It is the day that I begin the journey of weaving together into a cognitive and tangible format what has been bubbling around in me for a very long time. I have been gathering this content throughout my life and am excited to bring it together in the form of an easy-to-read book, that can instigate a gentle form of healing, of calm and coherence to serve you, the reader, and the people you touch, then ripple out into the beyond as a contribution to making our world a better place in which to live.

It is also a special day to me, in that on this day 93 years ago, my father was born. He took his final breath on February 21, 2016, which is exactly eight years prior to my final editing of this book, on February 21, 2024. I felt very blessed to be with him, along with my daughter, on his passing. My father was a kind and caring man. He was a hard worker and very much a family man. His family was the focus of his life. And the depth of his love for his children and grandchildren ruled his life.

Family gatherings were his absolute favourite events and seeing his descendants happy and healthy gave him so much joy. He was always so emotional and bursting with pride, watching the children as they sang in their Christmas concerts and reached their various milestones. I am proud to share this aspect with

him and do my best to keep all that he stood for alive within my family and beyond into our collective Universal family.

After his death, my life changed as an aspect of it dropped away and I had to navigate my way through some turbulent times, heightened by the grief at losing such an integral part of my life. Yet as one door closed, another one opened, and a sense of serenity filtered through and with it a new chapter began.

INTRODUCTION

Welcome to exploring my latest creation. This book is my gift to you in paying it forward. What does that mean? On my journey so far, I have been blessed to have been led to teachings, people and places who have helped and guided me, through the written word and beyond, to landing at this point I am in my life today. Now, it is my purpose through my written words to share some of my story, some teaching tips and practices that you can choose to incorporate and adapt as required, to bring about a stronger sense of calm in your life, then spread outwards to places near and far.

Thirty years ago, I wrote a book called *Changing the Paradigm.* The theme of this book was insight and tips on how we can change the paradigm, or world as a whole, to one that is more peaceful, wholesome, clean, clear, and prosperous. Yet, here we are, 30 years on, and from an outside perspective, our world seems to be heading in the opposite direction, in that wars are being fought, people are suffering, dis-ease is even more prevalent, crime is still happening, poverty, disharmony, and division are all around us.

This brings me much sadness, when I know that there is another way. I know in my heart that we can course correct and head out of this present state of chaos into one that is supported and held on a foundation of CALM.

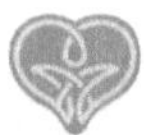

And like many of you, who will be drawn to reading this book, I pondered on what I can do as one small individual to assist in this course correction. And this book is part of my contribution. It was my intention to rewrite *Changing the Paradigm*, but after rereading and contemplating how to bring forward an up-to-date version, I am now choosing to start fresh, drawing from my life's experiences to create from the point in my life I now find myself. I will be sharing the wisdom I have gained from my ups and downs, wins and losses, and plenty of perceived failures, which is often where the most learning is derived.

This book will be filled with some deep spiritual insight, as well as some very practical tips on how you, as a seemingly insignificant individual, can BE the difference, to make the difference to function from that place of calm. I see so many good, kind, caring people around me seeing unrest, despair, unfairness, cruelty, and wanting to do something to make a difference, but don't know where to start. If you are one of them, then let me firstly invite you to see and honour your value and significance, then keep on reading, for in the reading of these words, you will also be receiving an energy of calm permeating within you.

You are about to be led through a maze of ideas and concepts to move through times of chaos, towards creating a life filled with more calm. When we have an inner sense of calm, we can navigate those turbulent times with more ease and grace, as if we are riding a wave of change with a sense of fun, rather than being pulled under, gasping for breath and being continually knocked about as if we are in a giant washing machine.

The first section of this book will start with looking at how we are all an aspect of Universal or Source energy, the importance of clear, energetic health and how language and parenting shapes us in a multitude of ways. This is followed by the importance of nourishing and moving our bodies in order to free our minds. The next section highlights you to where "rightness" limits your life and how to release it and connect to others in more meaningful ways. Then we move on to coming out of hiding, creating space for ourselves and using different techniques to free ourselves from old limiting patterns and programs into a more expansive space. Towards the end, I give you practical tips and tools towards creating more calm. If you are struggling with a sense of overwhelm and you feel like your life is in chaos, you might like to skip straight to the last section, then start fresh at the beginning again. Feel free to read this book in whatever order works for you.

Let me firstly introduce myself: I am a mother, grandmother, partner, teacher, healer, and friend, as well as being an aspect of God/Source/the Universe, as you are. I am here playing my part to the best of my ability in this game of life. I have always been a seeker, always looked and delved into more than meets the eye—always seen the bigger picture and had a deep insight into what is happening in this world. However, I have kept this part of me pretty well hidden and "close to my chest" in a quest to fit into a world I have never really fit into, in that a lot of my ideas and interests often don't really seem to align with the majority of people. I can see past what seems to present, into the vastness of our beingness, yet have previously shied away from sharing the fullness of all that I am and what is my Truth.

Now in my 60s after spending my entire life delving into and exploring spiritual principles, natural health, and personal growth, I feel that I have a lifetime full of wisdom and experience to share. This has come from not just learning, reading, and practising, but from a few hard knocks that life dishes out, some of which have contained the greatest droplets of gold. "I have been around the block a couple of times or maybe more."

My spiritual journey really began as a child, when I had an imaginary friend, who was a wolf, and interestingly came to life when I was 50 and my daughter drew her into physical form. Her name is Lydia and she has pride of place in my healing room.

Then, when I was in my 20s I found a book called *Dancing in the Light* by Shirley MacLaine. I devoured this book in record time, so excited to find another person in the world who also believed in reincarnation. In her journey that she shared, one thing that happened was that a book fell off a shelf into her hands. That book contained messages and wisdom that she needed to hear at that particular time. The next day, I was at the library shaking the shelves, waiting for a book to drop into my hands. It didn't; but I continued to scan the shelves for books on reincarnation and spiritual woo-woo stuff and there they were. I was beyond excited.

At that time, our local library was in the form of a bus and the librarian was a very cute young man who I secretly had a crush on and I didn't want him to think I was weird or anything, so I pretended they were for someone else as I shyly checked them out.

So many of us are riddled with a variety of fears and phobias, and the worrying about what other people might think of me is a big one. And probably one of the reasons it has taken me until now to share more of my message with the world.

As well as reading, exploring, and digesting the works and teachings of many of our great spiritual leaders, I have also been on and continue a lifetime journey of deprogramming, unplugging, and releasing old conditioning in a quest to find out more of who I truly am and why I am here on this Earth at this time.

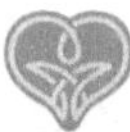

As you read these words and sense the energetic context in which they are presented, I invite you to feel into what is offered and take on board whatever resonates with you in this moment. Please explore further any topics or information that is of interest and do further research, if you would like facts and figures on anything that I share, as this is not my forte. Always be at the helm of your own ship and move forward from that place.

As captain of my own ship, I know that part of my role is to help and contribute, in whichever way I can, to alchemise chaos to calm in my life, and hopefully yours. If enough of us do this, then it will spread, until eventually we will live in a world where calm prevails. Sounds simple, and it is, and it's not. But what is simple is to make a start, go one step at a time, then keep on moving forward and let the momentum happen.

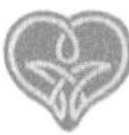

Chapter 1

ENERGY: OUR FIRST LANGUAGE

Do you know that only 5% of our communication is verbal? Yet 100% of our communication is energetic. Energy is our first language. At the time of our birth, we are an energetic being dropping into a human body. We are not born with language. We learn language, we learn everything we need to function in this physical reality. That is, how to act and how to live our lives. We learn from formal lessons and teaching, but most importantly, we learn it firstly from energetic interaction.

Everything and every interaction that we have as individuals has an energetic base. If we can read energy, it can help us interpret and move through life with that strong foundation of calm, in that we can sense either a space of calm or chaos in a person or situation and act accordingly. That act may be run for the hills or stay and play and learn.

Energy will always speak louder than words. This is really important in the area of parenting. Demonstrating how to act in a space of calm works much more effectively than continually telling or even yelling at a child how to behave.

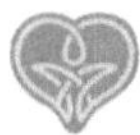

Have you ever walked into a room where you could literally cut the air with a knife? The energy is so thick that most people can sense something is amiss. Maybe someone has had an argument or heated disagreement? Or there is a big fat lie in the space being presented as truth?

Another example of energy that is not always so clear being transferred is after you have a meal. Cooking when in a bad mood or with lots of negative thoughts going through your head will transfer. I remember when I was a young busy mum, having a crazy day or upset or cranky about something, but had to feed my family and did it with the GRRRR attitude; this would transfer and next thing everyone would be fighting or grumpy. This was such a black and white example, yet it can happen with takeaway or processed food. Even in a classy restaurant where food is presented in such a beautiful manner, if the energy is not "clean" from the cook or maybe the waiter is having a bad day, any negativity will transfer.

I have been involved in lots of spiritual or healing groups, where people can be in a vulnerable and open state while healing or processing, and if that space is held in a loving and non-judgemental manner, it can clear easily, yet if people have any of their own judgements, opinions, or their own stuff in the way, making the energy heavy, then it can add to the person in their vulnerable state.

In a space of chaos, the energy is most distorted, yet in a space of calm, it is clear and crisp. That is where we want to head towards. Notice the sense of calm within nature? And around a new baby? He or she is born pure, whole, and healthy with a clear energy. Then compare this to a busy shopping centre. Or adults becoming heated and fighting over a referee's decision in a football match.

Animals communicate primarily through energy. My dog has been telling me for the past hour or so that he wants to go for a walk. I see it in his eyes. I sense it in his actions and movement. This is energetic communication. Animals, especially ones we have a close connection to, are continually teaching us in more ways than we may realise.

I was talking to a man recently about his dog. He was saying what a lovely calm dog she was, which I could pick up from her energy. During our conversation, he was sharing that she randomly went to attack a man once at a social barbecue. It was totally out of character, and they were very shocked. Later it was revealed that this particular man had been physically abusing his wife. Interesting how the dog had read the energy and acted out accordingly.

In the world in which we live, energetic connection between people is acknowledged to a certain extent, yet words, speech, and intellect are usually prioritised and sit at the top of the communication ladder. These aspects are important, but only if they match the energy with which they are delivered. Speaking a message of calm from an underlying tone or energy of chaos only creates more discordance and ultimately an extra layer of chaos.

Let me also clarify that when I refer to chaos, I am referring to it in its negative form, where it is out of control. Sometimes perceived chaos is actually elements rearranging towards a state of calm or neutrality. From this perspective, it is a natural part of healing and rebalancing. For example, when dealing with children, allowing a child to cry or tantrum can be what is required for them to rebalance back to a state of natural calm. Dogs will shake vigorously to rebalance their energies after anything that may interrupt their day or their sense of calm.

Chaos is not just an external force. It is, first and foremost, chaos within the minds of individuals. For in our world today it is this that "runs the show." What will that take to change? What will it take for energy to be our key language, with the words and actions to be formed and expressed from that energetic component?

Touch is another way in which we communicate. If that touch is not transferred from a calm or even neutral energetic space, then it is tainted. Touch can be very healing if it is transferred in this calm manner and can have the opposite effect if it is not. Even a massage or any form of bodywork or healing treatment could do more harm than good if the energy does not match the actions.

Generally, we have been trained and schooled and conditioned out of reading and feeling energy. My invitation through this book is to start retraining yourself to read the energetic component of a word, then a person or place or situation, and maybe adjust your conversation or interaction accordingly? How often do we simply go with the flow, rather than follow our own knowing or intuition?

So how do we strengthen and nurture our energetic health? What is energy anyway? It is not something we can see or hear or touch. It is something we can feel in varying degrees. What is our energetic health determined by? I believe that the easiest way to explain it is by the strength of our connections to God/Source/ Universe/All That Is/Quantum Field or that subtle guidance that we know exists. How pure is that connection?

Being in a pure state of presence is an indicator as to how fine-tuned our energy is, to all that we truly BE in our expanded state. In that space, our energy is clear and we are energetically aligned to our true self; the other 95% that we don't usually function from or tap into. Is that really possible, you may ask? That would be a desired state, yet how do we get to that place?

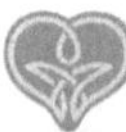

Chapter 2

CLEARING THE DROSS

In my experience, the only path to that pure state of presence and calm energetic space is to clear the dross; that is, clear what is in the way to being in that space. So how do we do that? This is where the fun begins. The journey is called LIFE. It is accepting ourselves in the purity that we know we are, even if we have never ever experienced it directly or cannot comprehend it with our mind alone. It is acknowledging that we are on this Earth at this time, living in this body to grow as a spiritual being and to find a connection to Source in doing whatever it takes to expand and grow that connection. This is a process, a continual process with lumps, bumps, and obstacles along the way. I refer to those impediments as "dross."

What if there is more to life than meets the eye? My understanding is that at the core of our being we are an aspect of God, Source, or the Universe. When we are fully connected there, we have the ability to merge with that energy and become as one with our creator.

From this place, we choose to bring this component of our true expanded self into physical form as a human aspect of God. We land in a body, which is not a random act, but something that is carefully chosen from our expanded state. I believe that we

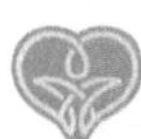

choose the parents and family and general path in life, which will give us the best opportunity to grow as the spiritual being we truly are and to have as much fun and joy as we can along the way. In this role, on this Earth plane, we function primarily from our physical, mental, and emotional states as well as our spiritual/soul/higher self, which is our unique energetic blueprint that carries us through all of our incarnations. The more we align and become one with this aspect, the easier it is to connect and be guided by Source/God/Universe/All That Is.

It is this expanded space that is the calm, yet as we begin our journey in our human form, we experience chaos, which is the dross playing out, often from a young age. In this instance, I refer to chaos from within our birth family; maybe Mum and Dad are together for the wrong reasons? Maybe the house we live in is a complete mess? Maybe we are born into poverty or a place of unrest? Mum and Dad will have their own dross as well, from their individual life experiences. Wherever we land, there will be some form of dross and as babies in a pure state, we will somehow pick that up and add it to our energetic field as we find our way in life. We will also pick up lots of love and clear energy from those around us. The ratio depends entirely on our circumstances. Maybe we also bring dross from our past lives?

Our job as humans is to clear the dross, deepen our connection to our higher self and ultimately to God or Source, so that we are guided from this space to live the best life we can in as calm a manner as possible; then spread this concept far and wide to create a world of calm and eventual elimination of chaos, as we know it at this time. Everything starts with us as individuals. The outside world we live in is a manifestation of our collective inner world.

From this perspective, I am hoping that you will realise the power and potency that you as an individual have to influence

and ultimately change what is happening in the whole of our world and our reality. Every thought that you have and every action that you take can have far-reaching consequences, without you even realising it. That is how powerful you are and how important you are in the big scheme of things.

"You are not a drop in the ocean, but the ocean in a drop"—Anandi Sano.

Let's delve a little deeper into clearing the dross from an individual perspective and even look at the concept of vibration. What is vibration? A vibration can be described as movement or shaking. Another description that I found is "A State of Being, the Atmosphere or the energetic quality of a person, place, thought or thing." This is what I am referring to when speaking about vibration.

When one's vibration is high, they have more of a connection to their expanded state and when it is low, that's when it is congested with dross. A general example of this is in a calm, serene place walking along the beach, we are in a high vibration as compared to maybe a crowded bus terminal when the buses are running late, are very crowded, and people are stressed, the vibration is usually low and the energy is full of dross.

I know that we have all felt the sense of serenity in nature, and being in such a peaceful place is conducive to calm, but not always practical and maybe even a bit boring to be continually in that space. We are here to live our lives, have fun, and to move at our own rate towards this state, no matter where we are and what is going on in our outer world.

At this point in time, there are a variety of events occurring around the world and possibly in your backyard. Be aware of the atrocities and natural disasters happening on our planet.

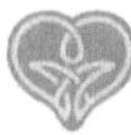

They are not something to be ignored and not something to be so focused on to the point that they drag you into a place of sadness, anger, and upset and keep you hostage there.

There are acts occurring that are "dehumanising" within the realms of war. Violence, crime, and cruelty are being perpetrated against our fellow humans in a manner that is not in any way aligned with our true nature. There are floods, droughts, fires, and cyclones that are affecting people in a horrendous manner. There has been a subtle, yet massive rise in artificial intelligence. We can see it and sense it and generally from our true human nature don't like or agree with it; yet it is happening around us more and more, so what can we do as individuals to keep those human aspects of kindness, compassion, and caring alive, well, and thriving?

I heard a quote recently that at the depth of our human suffering is a depth of love so great that it is all-encompassing and can override that suffering. This depth of love is a human quality. It is people caring for themselves and letting that high level of caring flow to others, in whatever way they can. This is what we have to awaken, acknowledge, witness, and celebrate to foster its growth, so it can multiply over and over. This may seem like a very tall order, amidst the high level of dross that is playing out and perpetuating the absolute opposite, but if you can step back, look at the big picture, and focus on the places, large or small, that love is working its magic, then anything is possible.

I am privileged to be witnessing this in my home state at the moment, where a large community has been gravely affected by a cyclone. In the aftermath, people are banding together, cleaning up the deluge and sharing what they have to those who have been majorly affected. My son has been involved in the repair and restoration to normality and in doing so, missed a special family holiday, which had been a long time in the

planning. This seemed almost insignificant to him after he had witnessed first-hand what others were experiencing.

There are enlightened people on this planet at this time, here to foster those loving, caring actions and non-actions. They have a very clear energetic space, which you will feel and ultimately have that state transfer to you by simply being in their presence, as they can hold a high vibrational field. There are also people who pretend to be enlightened and obviously, the opposite can happen in their space. That is why it is so important to raise your vibration so that you can perceive the difference.

I am sharing this information that may be feeling a bit heavy and even boring, but hang in there, as it is the foundation from both an energetic perspective and also an intellectual place. Please know that every word you are reading is encoded with a high vibrational energetic content, so by simply reading these words and soaking up the energy, a space of calm will envelop your being, which in itself is helpful in clearing the dross. Take your time, sit with this information, and allow the vibrational message to permeate.

Dross can create inner chaos, which can present itself as depression, anxiety, anger, despondency, stress, worry, sexual imbalance, overeating or drinking, or a general lack of clarity. Often, when we drop into these states, we can judge and beat up on ourselves even more. At that point, we can start to dissect it, try to fix it, work out the "whys and hows," or even take a pill or potion to make it go away or make ourselves so busy that we don't notice it anymore.

What if, when any of those negative states did arise, you took the time to stop, acknowledge how you are feeling, breathe, count to 100, possibly go for a walk or swim or move your body, however you feel to? Maybe even phone a friend who you

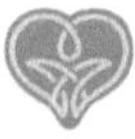

know will support you. Writing or journaling can be another good way to release those feelings onto paper. It is good to find an activity or practice that works for you, to bring you back to that state of presence and help you sustain it. I am hoping that reading this book is helping you in some way to BE in that present space and to truly acknowledge how unique and special you are. There is absolutely nothing wrong with you. You are not broken. You do not need any form of fixing. You are beautiful just as you are.

And you have a role to play in truly seeing the chaotic events that are occurring in and around your space and beyond, then delving deeply and seeing the loving, caring, kindness, and positivity in our world and focusing on that through your words, actions, and even thoughts. What will it take to bring these qualities to the forefront, so that eventually over time the negativity will have no footing and will have to fade away?

Have you ever heard the saying "What you focus your attention on expands"? I wonder if it could be true? I believe that it will take you and me as individuals to band together as a collective team to focus our attention on, shine our light, and whitewash that world of darkness and gloom looming over us from near and far. Sounds simple, I know. And it could be, if we could offload any of our own dross in the form of old conditioning, brainwashing, programming that we are carrying, whether we are aware of it yet or not, knowing that some of our dross has been passed down through generations, lineages, and beyond.

Be aware that clearing the dross is not an overnight process, but a journey—a journey that will have twists and turns, as we pass through a variety of scenarios. Some will be easy and fun and some may be challenging. They will vary from person to person,

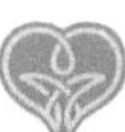

as we are continually presented with learnings in various forms. As we clear more and more, our vantage point continues to change and the bumps usually become less pronounced and of shorter duration.

Clearing dross is not a linear process. It does not have to be painful or drawn out or overly expensive. There are techniques and methods that you can learn and do yourself, as well as people who can guide you through a various array of practices. Everything you do comes from your own individual choice, which can vary and change, day by day or over longer time frames.

Let me intercept here with an example of clearing dross, if that is a concept that you are not familiar with. This instance was around clearing an old pattern of "people pleasing" that I know runs through my family, and maybe somewhere in yours too? I sense that I had picked this trait up from my mother's side of the family, which includes her mother and ancestors beyond.

Even though we often don't know and don't need to know their specific stories, we are all related and in an energetic context connected in some manner. So anything that I clear or that you clear can somehow clear a familiar pattern, which allows the next generation to be free from certain patterns which often can be causing pain or hardship.

I see "people pleasing" as a pattern of putting others before yourself in an attempt to keep them happy, often as a detriment to you keeping yourself happy, well, and of course calm, which is what we are working towards here.

My recent clearing was regarding a writing task that was suggested by someone more experienced that me in this field and made logical sense, but didn't completely feel quite right. I sat with it, trying to justify to myself why I should do it his

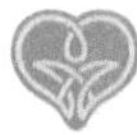

way, but just got myself into a place of confusion and self-doubt, so put it aside so as not to deal with it now.

The next day, I mentioned it to a friend and fellow healer and was guided through a relaxation session into a deep space of stillness, letting go of everything and everyone around me in that moment. As I sat in this space, I could sense that I was trying to do this task as per someone else's instructions, which were clear, but not quite me.

When I had this awareness, I took myself through a self-healing session and accessed a time when I was around 20 that the same pattern had arisen energetically. I knew it was all around "pleasing others before myself"; I could sense it and sit with it, then my body involuntarily shook and moved, before I once again settled into a place of stillness.

Later that day as I was driving, I got a clear message as to how to rearrange my work using a couple of the ideas presented to me, yet overlaying it with my own flavour. At the first possible instance, I took it out of the "too-hard basket," reworked the task at hand, and was happy with the end result. I felt more in my power after completing this assignment and use this as an example of clearing a clump of dross, as well as staying in my own lane and functioning as more of my true self and expressing accordingly.

Clearing the dross is also conducive to good health and healing. A high vibrational energy field free from dross is in alignment with a state of good physical and mental health, as well as a strong sense of self and deep inner knowing. When we are tapped into that deep inner knowing and allow it to guide us through our life, we will be led to people, places, events, and even books, classes, and courses that can help clear our dross,

create more healing, and ultimately balance in our lives, and with that, move towards accessing our true self.

Retrieval of Self

What happens as we clear the dross? We start to see glimpses of our self; that is, our true self. The word retrieval means to bring something back from somewhere and is of utmost importance when referring to our self and clarifies that we are already whole and healed.

We have simply forgotten or lost touch with those aspects, which would allow us to easily and often effortlessly live our most amazing lives as individuals and on a global scale. Our connection to that part of us has just been impeded by the dross we have been born into and created as we live our lives in a world full of chaos and fear.

As most of us are disconnected from this to some degree, I believe that as individuals we are in our human form to connect with and retrieve the aspects of our expanded self and bring them to the forefront of our present existence; that is, to see them more clearly and use them to guide us to a more wholesome, full, and fun-filled life.

In the clearing of our dross and retrieval of our true self, in essence, we need to turn ourselves and our world inside out, so that we see ourselves in our fullness, letting our lights shine brightly. This in turn contributes to switching on more light around us, which eventually can shine on the darkness, inviting it to be seen and acknowledged for all that it is, then run its course and eventually dissipate.

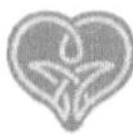

Chapter 3

INSIDE OUT—OUTSIDE IN

Imagine if we functioned from a space of opposites, as in, we functioned from love not fear, prosperity not poverty, clarity not confusion, and ultimately calm not chaos. Imagine if our media was full of acts of kindness, messages of love, and support for everyone. Imagine if our governments and associated institutions functioned from a high vibrational space where the energy of words and actions matched and were conducive to exposing and then clearing the dross, making way for real positive change towards more calm. Imagine if our health care system was truly focused on holistic health care rather than illness and drugs.

Imagine if our education system was focused on teaching children to truly honour themselves from an energetic perspective as well as developing the mind and body in a holistic sense. Imagine if our supermarket shelves were lined with fresh produce, rather than artificial, processed food. Imagine if there was no cruelty or war or starvation and people genuinely cared for each other in a loving manner. If we turned the whole world inside out, one person at a time, could we create such a world? That is the world I would like to see for my children and grandchildren and generations beyond them.

Collectively it could be seen as letting go of the old patriarchal reign that has held stronghold on us for such a long time and allowing the "enlightened female" to come to the forefront and lead the way. The world as we have known it, right back to earlier times, has been controlled largely by the energy of power-hungry and often cruel, narcissistic leaders. This energy of greed, force, domination, suppression of females, manipulation, control, judgement, punishment, and fear has been running the show for such a long time. And as a result of this, we can see evidence of this distorted energy playing out in the form of wars, chaos, starvation, cruelty, destruction, and poverty, somehow orchestrated by these negative forces at the helm.

Let me clarify that I am not talking about men and women here. I am referring to the male and female energies inherent in all of us. All aspects have a place and a specific role to play on an individual level and within the world as a whole. Often the Earth is referred to as Mother Earth as in the female energy and the blazing of the sun is often referred to as Father Sun which is more masculine.

Imagine if the female energy that has been ignored, suppressed, and punished in the past could be unleashed. What if the energy of kindness, caring, nurturing, equality, internal power, strength, and healing could come to the fore, in harmony with and being supported by the masculine qualities of logic, structure, physical strength, and power to begin to lead us all towards a world more aligned and balanced? Remember, everything is energy and energy can never die or disappear or be hurt or broken, but it can change form, reconfigure, morph, and shift.

To move towards this place of a more balanced energetic space seems like a mammoth task and it is, yet if everyone came on board, it would build up momentum and change could happen. The fear that is currently running the show would

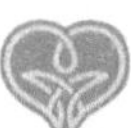

have to eventually subside and could be replaced by the true essence of love and energetic connection to our true self. This is not something that needs to be forced or pushed, but something that can happen organically with some genuinely loving support systems in place to guide those who are willing to do what is required.

I believe that this is happening in our world at this time as the dross is being released, corruption is being exposed, and more people are waking up to what is really going on. The dark places and fear-based activities are coming to the forefront in some places, as the world is turning inside out. What if we could see what was going on and do what is required on all levels to put out the fire, so to speak.

In saying that, we all have different roles to play. Some of us are there on ground level with a hose and water to directly extinguish the fire and some of us have a job to directly support those people putting out the fire. But the majority of people look on at such a situation in despair, wanting to help in some small way but not really knowing what to do and feeling helpless.

If that is you, and I know it is me, then what you could do is say a prayer, be in a space of stillness for what you can witness and are aware of, and send out the energy of love, from your own clear, unencumbered space. The clearer you are, then the more potent your flow will be. Everything that you do or say or think comes from you, the energetic space that you hold.

At this time, as our collective dross is clearing and we are witnessing some turbulent times, it is more important than ever to be the clearest, most expansive individual self that you can be for yourself, and ultimately our world. From the perspective that everything is as it is and life is unfolding as it is, things can appear relatively simple and they are simple from one perspective, yet not so simple at all from a different vantage point.

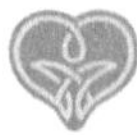

Chapter 4

THE POWER OF LANGUAGING

Now that you have got the picture and want to put your hand up to assist in making a change in your world and the world as a whole, let's get started with the nitty gritty. Let's move out of the space of procrastination and into action, whether that be physical, mental, emotional, or spiritual. Let's find some movers and shakers to get things really happening. Let's take some practical steps to clear the dross and retrieve and connect to our true expanded self, as we make our way towards creating and functioning from a space of serenity and calm, no matter what our outer world presents. Let's look into the words that form the language with which we communicate

According to the Oxford Dictionary, **procrastination** is the action of delaying or postponing something. But is it really the non-action or avoidance, either consciously or not? I have procrastinated on writing this book, not just for days or months, but for almost thirty years. Some people spend their whole life in procrastination, often sitting on the sideline passing judgement or making comment on those getting in and living their lives, boots and all. I am not passing judgement here, just noticing.

Let's firstly acknowledge procrastination for the role it has played in your life and mine and will continue to play, knowing that there is no right or wrong in anything. Everything is just a stepping stone towards a path of the retrieval of your true self. Some of these stepping stones present themselves as solid and strong, while others are wobbly and weak. Each of them has a role to play. Sometimes, they will give way beneath you and you will tumble and fall. And as you tumble and fall, you can stay down and stuck in the tangle of stories and excuses, regrets and the whys of all this, or you can hop up, dust off, and continue on your journey.

With each step, you are becoming closer to finding and accessing your true and sacred self. In finding that sacred part, could it be as simple as jumbling the letters to transform the scared self into the sacred self? One small shift of just one letter to lead to one big step into honouring the sacredness of who you truly be. Words as an entity hold such a powerful transformational essence. Look at the word **evil**, which when turned around the other way creates **LIVE**. Add a "d" to evil, then after a word jumble it shifts from **devil** to **lived**. Can you feel the energetic difference between these two words?

Discipline is something that we are conditioned to believe we need in order to eliminate procrastination or make some changes in our lives or certain behaviours. Take a look now at the word discipline. The dictionary meaning is "the practice of training people to obey rules or a code of behaviour, using punishment to correct disobedience." The word disciple means a follower or companion. What if we could become the follower or disciple of our God self and take energetic guidance, as it is presented? What if any change in behaviour could happen easily and organically, without any form of punishment? I like to substitute discipline with the word **devotion,** meaning "love, loyalty, or enthusiasm for a person or activity." Imagine if we had a sense of devotion for ourselves, how easily any change, from staying on track with an exercise routine or daily meditation, could become.

I invite you to look at words spoken in general conversation, such as **"this is killing me"**; **"that is sick"**; **"this is such hard work."** Whether words are spoken in jest or not, they all carry a vibration. I believe it is so important to be aware of the words we speak and use them in a positive manner. What if something could be **"healing you, instead of killing you"**? What if the **work is easy or fun,** or maybe sometimes challenging rather than hard? Can you sense the energetic difference in these couple of examples? Maybe close your eyes and feel the difference between the word killing as opposed to healing, between hard and easy, sick and well, and even chaos and calm?

Something that there is often a huge focus upon in personal development is goal setting. Let's look into the word **goal.** The meaning in the sporting arena is sending a ball between two posts or into a net on a sporting field, or within the area of personal development, what one would like to accomplish or attain. If you jumble the letters here, you have the word gaol, which is a place of confinement. I see a goal as something that can be very fixed and rigid, while our lives are continually moving, shifting, and changing, and know that many people get very disheartened if they do not reach their desired goal, to the point where they give up completely. In that light, I say leave the goal for the soccer field and in the personal development arena, substitute it with the word **intention,** which is an idea or plan to be carried out. To me, this gives room for movement and change, which is an adaptable component of life.

Another word that is widely used in the personal development field is **abundance.** The dictionary meaning here is a very large quantity of something. Quite often it is used in reference

to money or something that is favourable, yet unless that is specified, such as saying financial abundance, it could be a large quantity of bills or problems. My preference in this context is **prosperity,** which literally means being successful or thriving.

As we communicate, the brain works in a manner in which it initially hears a concept that is spoken and responds accordingly, then has to add any negative words to that idea as an add-on. In that light, let me suggest keeping conversation and especially commands or teaching in a positive format. As an example, a general conversation starter is **"How are you?"** and a general response is **"Not bad."** In that case the brain is focusing on the word "bad" and often the conversation moves on from there, down the path of the bad. An alternative here could be responding with **"I'm fine,"** which literally means of very high quality, which we all are. Imagine then letting the conversation flow along the lines of what is fine or good about you and your life. Remember, what we focus on expands.

A lot of people like to use positive affirmations, which when used in context can be helpful. **Expressing something in the form of a question** can also assist when looking to change or create something different or new in your life or to move through a hurdle that is causing concern. Questions can be a powerful tool in keeping the energy flowing. An example could be, if you have a presentation to do for your job that you feel nervous and unsure about, you could say, "What would it take to present my talk about frogs with a sense of ease and flow?" When using a question in this manner, we are not looking for an answer as that can stifle the energy. It is as if, we are putting our question out to the Universe and being open to any guidance we notice in regards to it.

Another example of **keeping wording positive** in teaching or parenting could be focusing on the behaviour you would like

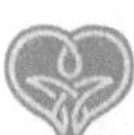

to encourage. You could say "**please walk carefully**" rather than "don't run on the concrete" or for a toddler "**let's do this puzzle**" rather than "don't play with the remote control." Avoiding the word "try" can help keep you focused on what you do or don't want; for example, rather than "I am trying to loose weight" to "I am eating more leafy greens in my diet and going for a walk each day" in that you are focusing on and bringing into the spoken word whatever is your intention. Avoiding "**try**" can make intentions more precise and clearer in that either you do something or you don't. How much time is actually wasted on conversation that dances around real issues?

Yet is a little word that can have a big impact. Adding it to any sentence gives it the scope to have something happen that you haven't created yet. An example could be instead of "I just can't walk up three flights of stairs" to "I can't walk up three flights of stairs easily YET," or "I haven't found my dream home" to "I haven't found my dream home YET." Anything is possible in any area of your life and using simple tools such as positive languaging and focus can go a long way.

Using the word **and** can give out the sense that you can have it all, rather than **either or**. If you are in the process of choosing whether to go on a holiday or do some renovations to your house, what if you can do both? Or on a smaller scale, within your day, rather than either getting a job done or going for a walk with a friend, what if you can do both? You can apply this to anything. The message here is that you can have it all, in every area of your life, and using AND in your languaging can contribute to acknowledging and creating all that you choose.

Be aware when living and creating your best life where you use the word **but**. When making a statement, using "but" to follow can be a precursor to an excuse, while "**and**" will add flow and momentum. An example here could be rather than "I would like

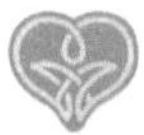

to go to this exercise class, but I have to wash the car," saying, "I am coming to this exercise class and I will wash my car later today." You can apply this to anything that is happening and let it add scope and expansion to any situation currently presenting.

Words are such a powerful tool, whether they are spoken out loud, written, or used in our self-talk. **Words have the power to hurt or heal**. Know or find out their precise meaning as well as feeling into their energy and use them wisely and with intention when sharing with others.

Words can also have a potent use in the form of journaling, which is another tool to release dross. If not appropriate to share in a certain instance, yet something is affecting you and stirring something within, then put pen to paper, then paper to fire, and let it all out.

Imagine if children were brought up with these patterns from a young age. Would they grow up as adults who could read any situation and act and speak accordingly, rather than following a direction that may or may not be conducive to creating a better life for themselves and then beyond? Where do we start with this process? I believe that we start with ourselves, with every person who would like to create a sense of calm and serenity within themselves, our community, our country, and our world.

From One Generation to the Next

As children, we learn from our parents from both their spoken and unspoken words. They, in turn, have learnt from their parents. Our pattern of communication is something that has been passed down through generation after generation, both consciously and subconsciously. I can recall as a young child staying with my grandparents, who I adored and wanted to do what I could to please them. They had a small hobby farm and had

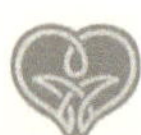

chooks to provide eggs. One day I was helping my grandma and was given the very important task of collecting the eggs.

I carefully gathered the eggs and placed them in a bucket to carry back to the house. As we were walking back, my grandmother was continually repeating to me, "Don't break the eggs." As a young child, my subconscious focus was on break the eggs, and guess what I did? The eggs came home broken and unusable and I was in trouble with my grandparents, but also was beating up on myself for being so clumsy for breaking the eggs. I wonder if my grandmother had said "Please be careful while carrying the eggs" in a calm voice, whether the outcome would have been different?

Spoken word often seems to be on automatic, as it was with my grandmother, as her parents would have most likely focused on a negative outcome in any given circumstance, as would have their parents done before them. What if now is the time to use our awareness, then to practise, continually focusing on what it is we would like to create, large or small in our lives? I believe this is something that can be changed and utilised to create more coherence and a greater sense of calm in our lives.

I grew up in the 1960s at a time when children were to be seen and not heard, where you did as you were told, or else, and went to great lengths to fit in and go with the flow. My parents cared deeply for me and loved me as best they could, as their parents did, and those before them. I was moulded and trained into being a good girl, not encouraged at all to look outside the box, as were many of us born in that era. Today, even though much has changed, the underlying patterns continue and the energy of control still has a strong hold on us, even though it is sometimes pointed from a different direction.

My upbringing was within the confines of the boundaries and conditioning of my mother, who grew up within the confines

of her mother, who lived within the confines of her mother, and back in time. I have spent much of my life untangling, breaking free, and knocking down barriers in my journey to connect more with my true, unencumbered self. Sometimes, I feel that the more I uncover and the deeper I go, the more obstacles I face. When the going gets tough, I often wish I had never opened that first door, but I did, and once open, there is no going back.

When I was growing up, I found it difficult to relate to my mother; I didn't like how I was treated and resisted as much as I could all that she told me to do on a conscious level. I could see, as I began to clear my dross, that I had subconsciously and unknowingly taken on a lot of her patterns and acted them out accordingly.

It is only in recent times as my mother has opened up more about her childhood and relationship with her mother, that I can see and understand more clearly, how she was also role playing the patterns that her mother had subconsciously taught her. Through each generation, each of us were doing the best we could within the circumstance's life had presented to us.

It is interesting as I look back I can see that I saw getting married as a safe and accepted way to leave home and move away from my mother and the control I felt she had of my life. Yet I unconsciously married a man who had lots of similar traits to her, which of course I didn't realise at that time.

I always find it fascinating that, as you unravel your own dross and unconscious conditioning, how you can see things from a whole different perspective. Today I have a healthy relationship with both my mother and my ex-husband and will always be grateful for the lessons they both taught me, the opportunities each of them gave me, as well as the positive and loving interactions.

I am especially grateful to my mother in demonstrating to me a variety of parenting skills, as her mother had displayed to her, some of which I passed on to my children and some I made a diligent effort to change, as well as lots of loving qualities from both of my parents and grandparents that I embodied and passed down to my children, and I get to witness them pass them on to their children as the cycle of life continues.

Chapter 5

PARENTING: A ROLE TO BE RELISHED

As well as acknowledging and being truly grateful for my early life, I made lots of deliberate changes from my upbringing in a variety of areas, in changing the way I brought up my children, as I began to clear the dross from my energetic field and perceive things from a different perspective. I also made plenty of mistakes along the way. Being a mum and now a grandma are the roles I cherish the most and feel honoured to continue to play. I believe that the role of the parent or caregiver can be one of the most underrated, underacknowledged, yet important roles we can play.

It is in this role that we have the opportunity to shape and influence the next generation of children into adults, who are energetically aware, kind, and caring towards themselves firstly and then others, and who live their lives with a strong connection to their true expanded self. It is a role that has influence on future generations and the direction in which the world and our lives will evolve.

Our mothering role actually begins when a baby is first conceived, then spends nine months growing within Mum's

body, being nourished by the food she eats, the environment in which she lives, as well as her thoughts, words, and deeds. After the child enters the world, the first nine months, she is still connected to Mum, now via her energy field. From nine to 18 months, she will gradually develop her own identity.

The greatest gift that you can give to a child as a parent or carer is to keep your energy field clean and clear, acknowledge your connection to your expanded/God self and actively do what you are led to, to clear your own dross. Anything you do for yourself will flow to your children and family as a whole.

When I was a young mum, I didn't leave my children much, so it was a big deal for me to leave my two-year-old to attend a self-esteem workshop. I was actually feeling a bit guilty for leaving her and her older brother, when the presenter delivered the message that being a parent with high self-esteem is one of the greatest gifts you can give your children. Your children will learn from what you do, not what you say. The younger they are, the better they can read energy and act accordingly.

Providing a comfortable place to live, healthy food and water, and a choice of activities and positive guidance as they move through the trials and tribulations life has to offer is also of utmost importance. Healthy boundaries are another key factor, as well as the power of saying "no," as difficult as it may be at times: this is all part of parenting and a powerful learning tool. Toys and trinkets are a bonus to keep in perspective, yet quality time in a state of presence is a true and wholesome gift.

Let me expand here on the saying no aspect. This is what creates boundaries for our children. These boundaries can be strong and healthy, wobbly and wishy-washy, full of gaps, or completely absent. The first would be my preference in creating an adult who is loving and caring, yet can say no with confidence and ease and walk away from whatever is not in alignment.

When I was a child, I was the eldest of four and played a role in mothering my younger siblings, especially my youngest sister, who was born when I was seven and a half. Our parents did a stellar job in meeting our physical and mental needs, yet had some room for improvement on the emotional side, so that was the role I played for my younger siblings. I was kind, nurturing, and playful with them, yet as a child, I didn't have the life skills or authority to say "no."

Many years later, after our father passed, I had to say no to something that was not aligned to me and didn't ring true. As a result, my younger sister exhibited the behaviour of a child having a tantrum because she didn't get her own way, which I know was her dross playing out, yet it got to the point where our family connection dissolved completely. To me, this is a classic example of the importance of saying "no" from a young age, so we develop skills to compromise and move forward in agreeing to disagree with any issue that may arise, yet still interacting with that person or people.

It is also a good example of "we are not our behaviour." The behaviour we exhibit is often coming from an accumulation of dross expressing itself when it can no longer be contained. This is why it is important to acknowledge and express feelings as they arise. When a child wants to cry, let them cry. When a child wants to speak, let them speak.

We all want to be heard and need to be heard. When this can be done in a safe space, in the moment it arises, the energy will stay clear. If our expression is stifled and suppressed, it will ultimately build up and come out possibly as inappropriate behaviour or, in extremes, possibly as illness, bearing in mind that there are other factors at play here, which include our environment.

Our environment includes the air we breathe, the water we drink, the food we eat, activities we participate in, people in our lives, and situations we are exposed to. All are relevant and it is important that we nourish ourselves in the most calm and loving way possible in all these areas.

Chapter 6

NOURISHING OUR BODIES: FOOD FOR THOUGHT, THOUGHT FOR FOOD

One area that I made some big changes in from my upbringing to that of my children was around the area of health and nutrition. When I was young, our meals consisted of meat and vegetables, some sweets, cereal, bread, vegemite sandwiches, SAO biscuits, a limited array of fruit, ice cream for a treat, and I can still remember having bottles of milk sitting in the hot sun for school morning tea. If we were lucky, we got a cream bun to go with it. That was the diet of the day and there was much merit to it.

My mother, who was born in the 1930s, was lucky enough to grow up with a father who was a natural gardener and they had a continual supply of fresh fruit and vegetables grown in healthy soil in their own backyard. She is now a healthy 91-year-old and I am sure her diet as a child has contributed to this. Processed foods were limited in those days and gym memberships unheard of. People got their exercise from hard manual work and such activities as chopping wood, walking, or bike riding to and from wherever they needed to go, maybe some old-time dancing, or a friendly game of backyard cricket.

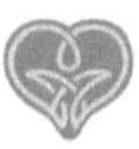

If you look at photos from that time, you will notice the women had hourglass figures, shown off by tailored fitting skirts and blouses, and men were usually very smartly dressed, Brylcreem and all. I saw an old photo recently of people crossing the road in Queen Street Brisbane in the 1950s compared to now. The earlier one highlighted the healthy look of the majority of people, whereas in the photo taken recently, most people were overweight and had a cup of coffee or can of soft drink in one hand and mobile phone in the other. That picture spoke a thousand words to me.

I wonder if people were really happier at that time or are they happier now with all the mod cons and such a high level of technology? There certainly seemed to be a greater sense of calm "back in the day." Life seemed to be simpler, people interacted directly with each other, and there was a greater sense of community.

Children built cubbies and played outdoors more, without the level of technology there is today. When my children were young, they had restricted TV time and I was aware of what they did watch, and I would like to think that today's parents do the same—keep computer and screen time to a minimum, monitor what they are exposed to, and encourage healthy outdoor play.

I know that we can't go back in time and there certainly have been a lot of improvements from then up until now. I, for one, would not like to give up the remote control that locks my car and opens my garage, or my dishwasher; but have we gone from one extreme to another? What if we could meet somewhere in the middle? What if we could see what did work from those times and incorporate them into where we are at now in our journey of evolution?

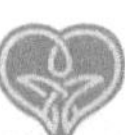

A couple of blatantly obvious changes that we could make could be cutting back on processed foods, and increasing homegrown fruit and vegetables, being aware that many of the minerals are no longer present in our soil and would need to be added manually. Having three meals a day is actually better for your body than continual snacking, as it gives it a chance to digest each meal properly before something else is added to our often already overloaded digestive system.

There are lots of simple home healing tips that can be incorporated into daily living when an injury or illness arises, before rushing off to the doctor for the latest pill or potion. The use of poultices, castor oil packs, cold compresses, essential oils, and the simple addition of garlic and ginger to our bodies, orally or through application onto the skin, can do a lot towards healing simple injuries and illnesses. When I was a young mother, I took it upon myself to educate myself in the area of natural health and healing and applied what I learnt within my family.

I encourage you as a parent or even a grandparent to do the same, so that you can pass down some simple practices to your children and down the line. I love seeing my daughter soaking garlic in honey to make a cough medicine and making a ginger poultice to reduce inflammation for a swollen ankle for her children. It also delights me to see my son growing fresh vegetables and fruit and the children picking them and enjoying these fresh healthy morsels.

Imagine if information on true natural health and healing was easily accessible and taught in schools or prenatal classes and more people became competent and confident in home healing. I'm sure it would free up our medical system for more serious injuries and illnesses.

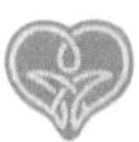

I have a little book called *Home Healing* by Margaret Wright, which was like a bible for me when my children were young. Barbara O'Neill has some amazing information on home healing and natural health, which is backed up by scientific evidence, for those who require it. I would certainly recommend listening to her work, learning from it, and implementing what you can, wherever you can, especially in regards to our most precious children.

Children's bodies are whole and pure, so feeding, nourishing, and healing them with whatever is most natural is most compatible to their growing bodies and developing brains. I always suggest keeping any form of processed foods, sugar, animal products, and breads to a minimum and keeping foods including fruit and vegetables that are as close as possible to their natural state in plentiful supply.

Many plants that we have classed as weeds are actually good for our bodies. The leaves on humble cobbler's pegs contain not only minerals, but also a very high protein content. The green leafy parts to many of our well-known vegetables such as cauliflower and broccoli contain much goodness. I take a walk around my garden each morning and pick leaves from varying plants in the yard, such as mulberry, kale, oregano, mint, spinach, blue top weeds, and cobbler's pegs, to create a yummy and nutritionally dense smoothie.

This is another area you can build up some knowledge in. I have a book called *Wildcraft* by Heidi Merika which has some valuable information regarding food foraging. Any food that is grown within your environment, which is the same energy field and therefore matches your energy as closely as possible, should be your number one choice.

And then there is wheat, which is very highly consumed in foods such as bread, cakes, and pastries, that we were brought up with and conditioned to enjoy. In the late 1950s, wheat was hybridised so that it would create a bigger crop, grow quicker, and feed more people. However, in this process, the composition was changed, in that the fibre and nutrients, including the bran and wheat germ, were removed. The wheat in earlier days was soaked, sprouted, and fermented, which also helped to remove some of the parts of the wheat that are unhealthy, such as lectins and phytic acids.

In the genetically modified version of wheat that we have been consuming since the 1960s, the nutritional value has been removed, leaving the endosperm which is the starchy part of the kernel that has little or no nutritional value and can cause sugar to spike, which can be responsible for various health problems we see today.

A synthetic form of folic acid has been sprayed on wheat in the US since 1993 and in Australia since 2009. Folate is a B vitamin occurring naturally in green leafy vegetables and conducive to good health, yet the synthetic form of folic acid has been attributed to detrimental health effects.

I was speaking to someone recently who had been living in Europe for the past two years, where it is not mandatory to spray it, and she was commenting that she ate and enjoyed lots of bread and pasta with no ill effects, yet upon returning to Australia could taste and feel the difference in these products. I wonder if this could be one of the contributing factors in the increase in allergies and intolerances to wheat products?

Overall, the wheat that we consume today is grown using synthetic farming methods such as the spraying of pesticides,

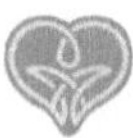

including Roundup which contains glyphosate. It has been said that wheat as it is today could be a major contributor to such chronic illnesses as diabetes, leaky gut, digestion issues, celiac dis-ease, and gluten intolerance, to name a few. Lots of reasons there to avoid or minimise the use of wheat or anything that has been genetically modified, taking it a long way from its natural state.

As well as what we eat, how, when, and why are as important to creating a greater sense of good health, nourishment, and energetic coherence within our body. The energetic components of a food which comes from the energy of the people who have handled it affects food intake as well. Your mood and where you eat and how present you are for your meal affects the energetic components, as in how it is digested.

It is a good idea to thank your meal and really acknowledge the components that have gone into creating it, just before you begin to eat. Being present and eating slowly and stopping when 80% full contributes to gaining maximum value from your food. Why we eat is another factor relating to food intake. Are you eating according to the clock rather than your body's hunger signals? Are you eating to fill a void that is really relating to another area of your life?

Fasting, and in particular "intermittent fasting," can also contribute to creating a greater sense of good health and wellbeing, in that it gives your body a rest from digesting, so it can focus more energy on healing and repair. Once you have been fasting for a period of 17 hours, a process called "autophagy" kicks in.

Autophagy is a basic cleaning out of old cells that are no longer functioning at maximum capacity, making way for new, fresh cells. This can be beneficial for improved brain health, hormone rebalance, weight loss, overall healing, and increased energy.

There is a lot of information available that includes scientific evidence as to how fasting is so beneficial to good health. Dr. Mindy Pelz has a smorgasbord of material on this subject.

Overall, anything that you put in your body, or on your body, for that matter, could create chaos or calm within, which roughly translated is dis-ease or ease within our bodies. Our skin is our largest organ, so whatever you apply to your skin soaks into your body. I suggest to take extra care and use your awareness before applying any product to any part of your skin. How close is it to its natural state?

Awareness is a big key in feeding your body and your mind. The stronger the connection to your expanded state the easier your awareness will guide you. The dictionary meaning for awareness is "knowledge or perception of a situation or fact." Again, the clearer your energetic space, the more fine-tuned your awareness would be. What if you just know, because you know in any given situation? Whether it be what food to eat or what skin products to use or to gain insight into any set of circumstances you find yourself in.

Water is something else to look at here, considering our body is 70% water. Not only is it important to keep our body hydrated, it is also important to be aware of what chemicals our water is laced with, which varies according to where you live. Then, if required, look into ways to filter out any nasties and possibly add some of the minerals that are in alignment with our body's composition.

In this light, drinking plenty of pure water is paramount to creating optimal health within our body. Most people aren't aware, though, not to drink water with food, as it dilutes the digestive enzymes, inhibiting the digestive process. Plenty of water between meals is the go and if you add a few grains of celtic salt to it, the pure water absorbs into your cells even better.

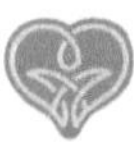

As a mammal, our body is designed to live to six times maturity. We mature at around age 20, which means in our natural human state, we are designed to live a healthy, happy, active life until around the age of 120 years old.

Unfortunately, at our present time, while most governing organisations are not being run from a place of energetic alignment to what is best for our bodies in the form of food and nutrition, it is up to us to create that sense of calm through good health; even though it may require extra effort and possibly extra cost, the results are worth it. If everyone made an effort to have more focus on healthy eating and optimum nutrition, then businesses that supported this would thrive and those that didn't, would either dissolve or transform into something more aligned to that space.

Chapter 7

MOVE YOUR BODY—FREE YOUR MIND

Movement is another powerful component to providing nourishment for our bodies, and creating more calm; while stagnation can create chaos within the mind, ultimately affecting the body. Movement is freeing. It can be used to release dross from the body and mind, therefore giving access to more of our whole expanded self. Movement, in alignment with awareness, is often termed aligned action, and can create amazing flow and magic within your life.

Movement can vary from a simple shake your body to a marathon run. It comes in so many different forms and modalities and can be used in any situation or place. It can be formal as in a sporting event or informal such as a walk on the beach. We have so many choices when it comes to moving our bodies.

When I am around children and they are niggling or arguing with each other and nothing seems to settle the situation, I will stop and sing and move to "Shake Your Sillies Out," inviting them to join. Usually, it defuses the situation very quickly and we all have a bit of a laugh and some sing and dance fun. And with all that, we have all shaken some dross away.

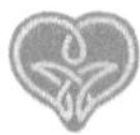

Stretching and gentle exercise, especially when done in sync with breath in a space of calm, is more powerful than it is often given credit for. Again, we are releasing dross from the body and clearing the mind in a really enjoyable and playful manner. Dance, whether it be in a formal setting or around your living room, is so freeing for the body and mind. I just participated in an online twerking party. This was something I had never heard of before, yet it was a bit of fun and focus on hip movement and as the instructor was so enthusiastic, it made for such an enjoyable activity.

Movement is really important to keep the internal workings of the body flowing freely and working to maximum potential. The lymphatic system plays a significant role here. It is paramount in keeping our immune system healthy by moving lymphatic fluid around the body, increasing blood flow to and from tissues and clearing toxins. We have major lymphatic "holding tanks" around the body, all of which are close to joints, so as we move our bodies and get these joints moving, we are also stimulating movement of the lymph fluid.

Manually stimulating these points can kick-start this process, heightening the benefits of movement. Dr. Perry Nickelston has a simple routine which I follow. In it, you massage around the major locations, starting at the collarbone, then behind the ears, under the arms, around the belly button, the groin, and behind the knee. I use this in my morning routine, followed by a short rebounding session.

Rebounding is such a great and simple activity. Benefits can include improving heart health by keeping the blood and other fluids flowing freely around the body. It is easy on the joints, may help in lowering blood pressure, strengthening bone health, and can even contribute to weight loss. Swinging on a swing in your local playground is also a fun activity to help move lymph fluid around the body. We are all different, so it is important to find what works for you.

This all sounds so simple and I know that most of us do some form of exercise, but how much do we prioritise it? Often, it is if we have time after all the other things we have to do that we might do some sort of a class or go for a walk or run or swim; then as it happens, time runs out and that couch with the remote control within reach looks just too inviting to resist and a pattern or habit starts to form. What if we could retrain to prioritise movement?

I offer conscious movement classes, which are a blend of yoga, qi gong, Pilates, and Feldenkrais, combined with breath work, presence, and the energy of calm. I love to see the change in people after spending just one hour moving their bodies and clearing their minds. I honour and acknowledge each person who comes to these classes. And I invite those who don't to consider it as a possibility or to find one that does work for you and make a commitment. It is taking the time away from the chaos and into the calm.

Imagine having these types of classes in schools and community centres all around, where they were even more accessible and even sponsored by authorities. Imagine the sense of calm that could spread all around. I wonder, if the focus was a variety of movement activities, conducive to clearing the dross from a young age, whether people would have a greater sense of good health and a stronger connection with their expanded God self.

There are so many forms and variables of movement available at this time. It is important to find whatever works for you and fits into your lifestyle.

Let me stress here the importance of doing movement or exercise that is in line with what your body requires, not what

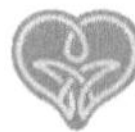

you think you should do. Like everything, there is the other extreme, where people are overexercising in an activity that could possibly be detrimental to their health and can create dis-ease or dis-harmony within the body. Movement is not necessarily about going for it gung ho. It is about finding what works for your unique body and choosing from that place. I have a little saying that anyone who has been to any of my classes will be familiar with. It is to Continually extend your Comfort Zone, but never to push into any pain.

Any form of pain in your body is your body speaking to you. The message usually starts as a whisper and can progress into a scream, if ignored for long enough. Sometimes your body may be telling you to stop and rest or to change direction, into doing something entirely different, or maybe take a break for a period of time before returning from a space of refreshment.

At times your body may be asking for some sort of treatment, which could range from a massage, maybe chiropractic, physio, acupuncture, osteopathic, craniosacral, Bowen, or maybe a visit to the doctor. All of these modalities and a lot more can help release energetic dross that is stuck in the physical body. Sometimes one person may have wonderful results from a certain treatment, yet someone else may not, so once again I encourage you to find what works for you at any given point in time, knowing that your cells are continually replenishing themselves and your body is continually working to bring itself to a state of optimum health in every moment.

When choosing a treatment, firstly look at the practitioner. The more present and clear this person is, the better your body will receive and respond to any treatment. It is such a gift when someone is working with you, that they are focused on your body and what is presenting from a state of presence. If you find someone who is not focused and maybe checking their phone, telling their own stories, or being distracted in any way, that could be a red flag.

I had a perfect example recently of being led to a practitioner who I hadn't been to before. I had seen a sign advertising for acupuncture. I hadn't had an acupuncture treatment for over 10 years, but this was the reminder I needed. I looked up this place, and was scrolling the ones in my area. I landed on one who had appointment availability which suited perfectly.

I did have some acupuncture in this session, but it was the bodywork that this practitioner also practised that my body required. As he touched a spot on my hip, I felt a wave of nausea and started coughing. I knew this was some dross in the form of stuck energy releasing. After the treatment, I felt so tired and needed to have a short rest in a state of presence for a bit, to allow it to somehow integrate, before I got up and continued my day. I share this experience as an example of "clearing dross." I had not gone into this session with that intention, yet it happened instantaneously, under the appropriate circumstances.

Our bodies are made up of trillions of cells and are always upgrading. New cells are continually regenerating or old ones could be looping. New neural pathways can be forming, while old ones release. Our body is an amazing intricate aspect of who we are and is very much affected by our energetic state. It is capable of being in a calm state of bliss or a disruptive and chaotic state of dis-ease and dis-harmony, or somewhere in between. I believe that it is our body's natural desire to be in a state of good health and it will do whatever possible to move towards that state. Every signal that we get is lovingly guiding us there.

So why do we see so much ill health and bodily discomfort? Could it be that we let our minds, that are usually very congested with dross in the form of negative self-talk, affect our body in some way? The first step to changing this is awareness.

Chapter 8

AWARENESS: THE INVISIBLE THREAD

Awareness is a key that winds its way through all of these chapters, yet deserves a whole chapter of its own, to highlight its role as the link to bind so many steps together to create a smooth and gentle flow. Awareness is an integral aspect of returning to our natural state of calm and ultimately good health within ourselves and beyond. Awareness is firstly acknowledging the chaos or whatever is presenting for what it is, without any judgement, then it allows you to drop into a state of acceptance. Let's delve a little deeper into acceptance.

The meaning of acceptance is "a person's consent to the reality of a situation, recognizing a person, process or condition, whether it be positive or negative without attempting to change, rectify, judge, resist or protest it." When applying to one's self, it is embracing and honouring every aspect of ourselves. Self-acceptance is an integral part of deeply acknowledging the place you are standing right now and from that place moving towards a calm acceptance of others. It is only from that space that a graceful movement has the potential to spread that state of calm in all directions.

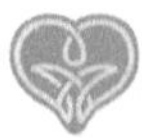

This may sound simple, yet when we are being run by the continual looping patterns of our dross, it can be hard to distinguish between what is real and what is programmed in both our personal lives and what we see in our environment and across the whole of the world. How much do we align and agree with a point of view just because it is drummed into us over and over?

This is how advertising works. We see a concept over and over and eventually we buy it as real and true, and the story continues. Hearing a concept repeatedly actually pushes it into your energy field until you will often take it on. This concept can add to the dross and be used to create more chaos or it can contribute to releasing some dross and creating more calm. Can you see this in the light of media reports? When we have something told to us over and over and we are not clear in ourselves, we can easily take it on board as our own point of view. However, if we are calmer and clearer in our energetic field, we can be more discerning.

Imagine if we were continually told by outside voices how amazing and wonderful we were. We would eventually believe it, especially if everyone around was hearing and believing it too. Music has a powerful effect here. It can be a powerful tool for clearing some dross and uplifting our mood or can have the opposite effect. I used to play positive affirmation music to my children when they were young and feel that this can be great to use as a parent or teacher to move us towards more positive self-talk.

And for yourself, when one of those catchy tunes goes around and around in your head, change the words so they are positive and uplifting. Here is one of my favourites that I sing out loud or silently, depending on what else I am doing.

"I am Love, I am Light

 I am Universal Sight

I am Love, I am Life, I am Power."

It is so simple and always uplifting. Choose your own tune and let it loop!

Imagine if we had awareness around what to consume. Could we create more serenity and calm in our minds and bodies? The dictionary meaning of consume means to "devour, take in or use up," so consumption could be in the form of food, environment, music, TV, movies, even interaction with those around us. Everything we are in connection with, we have the possibility of consuming.

That could be with any of our senses. We can consume the sweet fragrance of a rose or the strong smell of petroleum. We could consume fresh healthy food or a quick processed take-away. We could consume the energy of witnessing a crime or the serenity of a peaceful sunrise on the beach. We could consume the healing power of crystal bowls or some deafening sounds that can have the opposite effect.

None of this is right or wrong. It simply is what it is. Right or wrong or good or bad or winners and losers: all come from judgement. Is there any judgement when we are functioning from our expanded self? I think not. Judgement again is a part of the dross that we have created. Imagine a world without judgement. You may say that we need judgement to decide winners and losers.

We live in a world where winners are celebrated, and rightly so in most instances. But what actually makes a winner? One could say it's a whole lot of losers. What if the real winners are

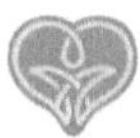

those behind the scenes doing the inner work in clearing dross? What if winning could be an inside job? What if you are a winner because you woke up today?

Imagine if there was no formal competition, and all activities were created to simply have fun. Imagine if nothing was better or worse than anything else. Everything was just different, including points of view. Imagine if all people were acknowledged and honoured for their differences, instead of ridiculed or even abused. Imagine if we could align with people that not only had a matching point of view to ours, but also had a differing opinion.

Chapter 9

IMAGINE A WORLD WITHOUT RIGHTNESS

Is it right to be wrong or wrong to be right? Rightness is where you are so focused on your point of view that you cannot perceive anything else. We often label people as stubborn, who are so right about something, nothing can seem to budge them from this place. To have rightness, we must first have judgement.

Let's look more deeply into the subject of judgement, from which rightness is derived. I found this meaning "the process of forming an opinion or evaluation by discerning and comparing." In a neutral space, judgement seems harmless and can have its place. Yet in reality, it can have some very negative connotations, in that it can chip into and erode healthy self-esteem and create hurt and upset and very often, some deep and difficult-to-detect chaos.

The most damaging form of judgement comes from oneself and once taken on and set, it can loop over and over and intensify, creating more damage and destruction, if left to play havoc with our mind. When we have a deep sense of calm, down to the very core of our beingness, which is found through our connection to our God self, then the judgement cannot land

and will fade away. This is what we are moving towards as we clear our dross.

However, part of this process is being aware of the judgement we have towards ourselves first and then others and use whatever process that works to clear and release it. Once it takes hold, then a pattern can form across many levels and may need to be released from different angles and perspectives. That is why clearing dross is a process. As we move through this process and things shift, we will feel better and calmer, no matter what our external circumstances present. Sometimes though, we can drop into our old patterns again, without even knowing it. This is where awareness is required to do more clearing and shifting towards more of that energy of calm.

I know that I have jumped into my dross and instigated blame and regret when my thinking mind tells me that I have already cleared this, using all those techniques I have learnt. The techniques must be wrong and the people that teach them must be wrong and everything just sucks and I am on the treadmill of self-loathing once again. I have often fallen into this trap and wallowed around in it, feeling sorry for myself, so focused on the rightness of my point of view and wrongness of others, that I become stuck again in procrastination and inactivity. Can you relate?

Rightness can have such negative consequences and be responsible for creating much dross. I can still remember one incident as a young child in a primary school maths class, where we were given a problem to solve. I came up with the correct answer, but had not used the right method, so was in trouble for that straight away.

While we were doing this task, I was helping my friend while the teacher wasn't looking and of course our answers and methods were the same, which we would have got away with,

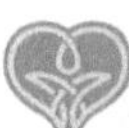

except for my unique way of arriving at the answer. Because of this, we were both pulled up for cheating, hit heavily across the head, and made fun of in front of the class.

The shame I felt was not just for me, but for my friend, who received the same punishment. This scenario all stemmed from the unwavering rightness of that teacher as to how to do each step of this particular mathematical problem. Imagine if that teacher had praised me for finding a unique way for coming up with the correct answer and for helping a friend, who struggled in this area.

Another time when rightness was playing out, was when I was driving to an event, running a bit late, and was continually told by my passenger that I was going the wrong way and that his way was better and would get us there quicker and easier. I knew that my way was right and he knew that his way was right. The scenario caused much upset for both of us, yet in hindsight, we both had different routes to get to the same destination; neither were right or wrong and if one of us could have calmly listened to the other person and done what was best for us in that moment, much angst could have been avoided.

Rightness can cause argument and upset in relationships, ranging from a casual friendship to a deep, intimate relationship. When I separated and ultimately divorced after 30 years of marriage, I initially found every bit of wrongness about my husband and was so right about it. It caused much upset for both of us.

In hindsight, when I was eventually in a place of neutrality, I could see that our relationship as a couple had run its course, caused by no right or wrongness from either of us. In time I could see clearly the treasure from those years, as well as mine some valuable lessons, which I could use in all forms of future relationships.

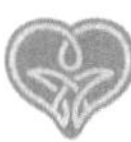

I invite you to look at the part that rightness plays in your life. I see rightness almost as a "dis-ease" of this time and something that certainly contributes to the chaos in our inner and outer world. Not just plain rightness, but rightness of a point of view. Where is it that you are so right about something that it actually brings a tightness into your body and stuckness in your mind?

I know that I have certainly functioned from a level of rightness around a point of view, often the rightness of a point of view that was not even mine in the first place. I have allowed myself to take on the opinions and teachings of others at the expense of disconnecting to my own truths. I have been led down rabbit holes only to resurface in a vulnerable and wobbly state and fallen down once again.

I have ignored and downplayed the gifts I was born with and resisted my path and my reason for being. I have channelled my energy into projects, courses, and teachings that really didn't serve me and have become complacent, despondent, and even self-loathing. I have allowed my conditioned self to run my life. I have spent a lot of my life swimming and sometimes drowning in the chatter of my mind. I have been so full of dross that I haven't been able to "see the forest for the trees."

I have given my power away to different sets of "theys." I have had such a rightness about the wrongness of the world in which we live, that I have resisted the practicalities of my life and what was going on in the world and instead turned to spiritual teachers and self help gurus. I thought they must have all the answers and put them on a pedestal, then allowed myself to be brainwashed and tried to become someone I was not. I have let the opinions of others override my own. I have almost lost connection to my true expanded self that I was searching so hard to find. Then I

have beaten myself up again for ignoring those red flags and not knowing better. I have let fear and anxiety shut me down even further.

All the while maintaining an outward expression of it's all okay. I am okay. I am focusing on the positive. There are people worse off. I have a lovely life. At the same time, continuing to search for yet another modality or teacher or guru who would be the one. Could this be the course or technique I need to feel amazing all the time? To have crystal-clear clarity on my direction in life? And I would always find something and feel better for a bit, then crash again.

Yet all the time knowing that there was more to me, more to life than I was experiencing and participating in. My search continued. One of the courses that I did during this search was life coaching. I excelled in the practice sessions that we did using the techniques we learned as a life coach and once I even received a standing ovation for my coaching skills. Yet in the area of marketing and promoting myself, I failed miserably.

One marketing activity we had to do was go into a busy shopping mall, stop people in the street, and sign them up for coaching sessions. This was way too far out of my comfort zone, so I went and hid in a public toilet and made up a list of imaginary names, then snuck out at the assigned time and back into the class. I felt so bad and wrong that my self-esteem slipped miserably once again. Now, years later, I can laugh at this scenario.

What I noticed in this arena, was that the people who excelled in promoting and selling themselves and their business were the ones who were out in the world doing this job. Amongst these people were some amazing coaches and practitioners, as well as some who were and still are, doing this personal growth

and healing work from the energy of power and greed and functioning from their own dross. Yet they are so right about what they are doing, people seem to follow them.

Rightness can extend past us as individuals as we form friendship groups or cults, all with a matching rightness around a point of view. This can grow to very large proportions. In previous times and even now, we see this in religious groups. There has been a certain exodus from a lot of religions and into different spiritual modalities and groups, most of which began with some beautiful, clean, pure teachings from that expanded self, connection to God from the original teacher. Yet the dross of the followers can often congeal into a strong sense of rightness, which can distort the original teachings.

How do we tell the difference between organisations, teachings, and practices that advocate ways and techniques to clear your dross and heighten or sharpen your connection to your own expanded or God self? We use awareness. Awareness has the ability to override rightness. Awareness is the first step in perceiving where you are so right in certain areas and about certain people or ideas, in that you have such strong and fixed opinions, that there is no room for calm or a sense of serenity, and making some changes from this viewpoint.

The other aspect of awareness is to be clear that it is your own unique awareness; that is, to "stay in your lane," as such. Sometimes you have to step away from a situation to see it from a larger perspective. This is also important in personal relationships. I believe that, even in intimate personal relationships, it is good to continually refresh them. Sometimes you even need to pivot or step away completely, regroup, reassess, then consciously

choose to step in again, or not, from the same angle or a totally different one.

And this is a key in any friendship groups, spiritual organisations you are a part of, or even political parties, sporting groups, or clubs you may be affiliated with. Continually step away, find your own footing, regroup, then choose to step in again, if it is still aligned with who you truly be and the energetic connection is clean and clear. If they do not support you to do so, then this could be a red flag for you to notice.

I was involved in a personal development modality for many years. I went to many classes, spent a lot of money, practised their techniques, and listened to their teachings over and over to make sure I got it right and got my money's worth, interacted and was friends with others who were also involved here, had some fun and laughter and tears and upset, and revolved my life around their teachings. I had some red flags along the way, but feeling such a sense of belonging made me override them all.

Eventually I did step away, then slowly over time, begin to untangle and disconnect and see what really wasn't working for me and probably never would. I also had to extract the aspects that did work for me and the great learning here. And there are some of these tools, techniques, and teachings I still use today and some friends that I made at that time that I continue to keep in touch with, yet most of it I had to let go completely, then clear a lot of dross that I had accumulated during that time.

In sharing this, I do acknowledge that we do need teachers, coaches, techniques, courses, books, and friends to assist us on our journey towards finding our own calm, heightening and fine-tuning our own awareness, and creating a fun-filled life along the

way. And we do need connection. Every experience I have gone through has made me the person I am today, which is something I am truly grateful for and something I hope you can relate to.

On a larger scale, we can see much rightness in the political arena, sporting groups, and religious organisations. Some spectators are so right that their favourite team is better than another that it can lead to physical violence. Often political parties or whole countries are so right that their ways, systems, and policies are better than anything else that they go to great lengths to prove it. Could all this contribute to fighting, wars, and unrest around the world? I know that it seems like we are such a long way from shifting this, but I believe that the willingness to be aware of how rightness plays out and perceive life from a different perspective could go a long way.

Chapter 10

FINDING THE GAP IN THE FENCE

Let's now drop any of our rightness, take a breath, and look at life from a different perspective. Let's expand our outlook and feel into more than meets the eye and then lean into it, taste it, and even drink some of that delicious nectar that is freely available from this vantage point. Is it time to find the gap in our own self-imposed fence and explore this concept? Is it time to take a journey to this space?

I invite you to imagine that we live in our own world, within our own self-imposed box or bubble, that we have fenced off in some way. This fence has been created by us, by our conditioning and our lifestyle, and this fence creates a sense of safety for us to function, in our day-to-day lives. Within this fence we create our environment, our comfort zone. We can decorate it to our liking, use our creative instinct to make it our own, then change it according to our mood or the flavour of the day, month, year, or years.

Within this space, we can dance and play and move in whichever way we please. We invite whomever we choose, into our space. We can be happy or sad in our space, but know

that whatever mood takes us, we are safe to express ourselves. We can move around and let this space move and expand and morph into whomever or whatever we would like to be in any given moment. We can live our entire life in this space and be happy. We can even clear our dross in this space and then clean up the mess. We can see people come and go in this space. We can adventure and see the world from the safety of our own unique space. And we can die in this space.

So how do we create this space in the first place? Is it something we are born into? I believe that our parents invite us into their space when we first take on our physical form and begin our role as a human on this planet at this time. The main job of our parents is to keep us safe, and from this place to nurture and mould or shape us into healthy, happy people, about to live our best lives. Then as we grow up and mature into adults, we also create our own space. It may overlap with our parents and birth family, or it may not.

And the cycle continues, with each of us in our own safe space, which we live in for the whole of our lives, decorating it with our own stamp, having fun, navigating the ups and downs and riding the waves of freedom, all within our bubble. If the movement gets rough, then we can tighten our space and drop even more into our safety net and when we feel flowing and amazing, with a sense of freedom and adventure, then we can expand this space again. And because it is primarily created from "energy" it will comply with ease.

But what if there is a gap in the fence around our place? Can we see it? Can we sense it? Do we know it is there? Would we like to go through it and venture outside our safe, comfortable space? Could it be safe to squeeze ourselves through or would we most likely get stuck, maybe even cause an injury? And why would we want to venture or even peek through this gap in the fence? Our life is happy from where we are. We have learnt to deal with the wobbly bits. There is a copious supply of Band-Aids and spakfilla in our space. There are various checkpoints here with an endless supply of lotions and potions to make us feel better, if we need them. And we have all of those anonymous "theys" to help us out when required. They are our friends, after all, there to watch over us, keep us even safer than we could ourselves, so why would we ever want to shift from this space?

We have all the trinkets we need here, and there are always more, at a price of course. And so many other people live in their own space and are happy and content and lots of those people are our friends. They like us and we like them and we look out for each other. We help keep each other safe, then, if ever our safety is compromised even further, the "theys" will step in and come to the rescue. We can always rely on them.

What if we did venture out of our space? The first step would be to find and access that gap. It is almost like finding a "needle in a haystack" or in a recent experience I had, "finding a pendant in a forest," when I was walking my dog through the bushland near my home. The day before, I had purchased an EEmedalion for him and tied it to his collar. Just as we were about to get back in the car, I noticed it was gone, so it must have fallen off somewhere along the track. Now, this was not a one-path track. I turned him around, trying to remember which path we had taken, but kept getting more lost and confused as to where we had been; however, I was determined to find it. Eventually, we went back to the start point, retraced our whole route and there it was, sitting amongst the leaves, only just visible enough to retrieve.

What if this is a similar scenario to finding the gap in the fence, yet this one is in an energetic format? It's about being determined to find it, knowing it is of value, then keeping on looking no matter what it takes. And this is a choice. Some

people are happy to live their whole life or lives within that fence, and some of us would like to slip through that gap and see what is on the other side—look at life from a different perspective. And what if it is there that the magic lies?

What if you can see things from a different perspective from this place? What if this is the place where calm prevails and life is lived from this foundation? Choices are made from the space of calm. The safety is still there, but set from a different angle. This is where the world is inside out from that of the bubble. It is much clearer. People here are continually clearing their dross, but now it is dispersing into the vastness of this expansive space. Everyone can speak their truth and are seen for who they really are in their expanded state. They take full responsibility for their life as an individual and in the connection to the whole big scheme of things. Chaos is still present, but seen in a different context as if it is now a catalyst to pivot back onto that path of calm.

There are still individuals with different points of view in many different areas; however, now these are acknowledged and accepted. Everyone is honouring and supportive of wherever each other is at on their journeys and of each individual's talents, abilities, and purpose in life, none being better or worse or more or less prestigious than another.

All life forms in this space are treated with care and respect and accolades when due. There is such a sense of fun and laughter here. Song and dance and movement practices are at the forefront of activity and mishaps are treated in a place of healing from all directions, with the energetic guiding the

process. There is no force or push or shove, just freedom and flow. There is ceremony for life's milestones and each phase of life is acknowledged and celebrated.

There is a sense of heightened awareness. Community is prevalent here and people work and play in their chosen role, each contributing to each other in whatever way they can. Differences and problems do arise, yet are sorted and worked through towards a mutual collaboration. The wisdom of the elders is honoured and respected. Each individual has their unique role and does it joyfully, and together people and their surrounds unite in a calm space with a sense of serenity.

And from this perspective, it is easy to see what is going on within people, community, countries, and other worlds and choose to interact and continue to live in that space, travelling with ease now, through the gap in the fence, into the beyond and back again.

As more people find their own "gap in the fence" and go through it, it opens up and invites more of those who are still clinging to the safety of their old spaces to expand and explore what is beyond.

My invitation through this chapter and the energetic transmission within it, is to start to explore and find the gap in your fence and mosey on through. This in itself will loosen some of your dross and it will fall away as you float into the beyond. As you settle into this expanded space, your energetic field will expand and your connection to God/Source/Universe/All That Is will strengthen.

Chapter 11

HEALING THE HABIT OF HIDING

Healing the habit of hiding and the dross that is keeping it in place is a prerequisite to finding the gap in the fence and exposing your true self, in whichever form that presents in this moment.

I just got a visual of a support group for hiders and I am in it, sitting in our share circle, ready for my turn. I pull up my big-girl pants, stand tall, and introduce myself. "My name is Helen and I like to hide." Sounds a bit weird, I know, but that would be a big, brave step for me, even more so in my younger days. I share this chapter with any fellow hiders, friends of hiders, or those who have a hider within their family, and those who don't even realise that they are hiders, which was me.

Upon reflection, as a child, I hid behind my mother's skirt. I have hidden behind my siblings, my husband, and even my children, all because I always felt they were better than me, more successful, had a better education, more sporty, more capable, more sociable, more tech savvy, or more attractive. I grew up with a not-good-enough, don't-really-fit-in, nobody-likes-me-or-even-notices-me outlook on life. So hiding was a good option and one that I became really good at. It served

me well, in that I settled into my comfort zone, focused my attention on my home and my children, and lived a nice life.

As I did this, I always found a way, through a book or a course or interaction with like-minded friends, to satisfy my obsession with personal growth, spiritual healing, and all things weird and woo-woo. Those around me often made fun of all my "crazy stuff" but I just laughed it off. I practised different modalities and did what I needed to do to keep myself and my family healthy and well along the way, so long as it was in the parameters of my own safety and most importantly, that of my family.

In the 1990s, my go-to place was called "The Inner Energy Centre," where I would go each week with one of my babies in their baby basket, asleep alongside me, and I would receive a hands-on healing, then sit in a solitary room and meditate. I did this, year after year. It was a safe space for me. I felt accepted as I was.

Around that time, I had two special friends and we would meet in person and do healings locally and universally, all within school hours, of course. They brought forward a meditation program called ISIS meditation, which I contributed to, and we used it to guide and heal people in what I refer to as clearing your dross. I then wrote my own program called "Corinthisis," which also helped in this process.

It was during this time that I wrote my earlier book, *Changing the Paradigm*, which I self-published, then sold and gave away, maybe a couple of hundred copies, and was quite proud of this achievement that I had created at that time, when I had a two-year-old, a teenager, and two children in between. And I received some positive feedback from people, even going so far as to say it had saved their lives, and I also received some

negative feedback from people who had been triggered by some of the concepts introduced.

Instead of taking all of it in my stride, I took the negative comments to heart and went into hiding once again. I stopped writing after that and turned my attention to studying homeopathy, which I could use in my home healing cabinet and still use to this day. I loved this modality and ended up working in a clinic with it, many years later. Another great hiding place?

Hiding behind your pain can also be a very subtle and sneaky hiding place. That can happen when people focus so much attention and live their lives around the pain they are experiencing and what is wrong with them, that they limit their lives immensely. I am not saying here to ignore pain and not acknowledge the severity in which it can present. I am saying to keep it in perspective and prioritise your focus on what you can enjoy.

As I share my hiding experiences with you, I clear some more of that dross that is preventing me from exposing myself more and more. What is it that I have been hiding? What is it that you have been hiding? Is it your greatness, your brilliance, your skills and talents in one or more areas? Is it the fact that you are an amazing parent or grandparent, wonderful friend or partner, fantastic pet parent, kind and caring teacher, helpful son or daughter, or maybe a great worker in your chosen field? We all play a multitude of roles. Do we acknowledge ourselves for what we do in these roles? Do we acknowledge ourselves for being the best person we can be at this point in time, with the knowledge, skills, and abilities we have accumulated during our lives?

Let me acknowledge you for reading this book and allowing it to guide you. Let me acknowledge you for accepting the point that you are at right now and for either taking steps towards

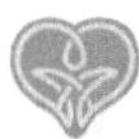

clearing your dross, or the stuff you have already cleared. Let me acknowledge you for your brilliance and beauty. Let me acknowledge you for living your best life. Let me acknowledge you for the kindness and caring you display towards yourself and others. It is all relevant in making the world a better place. And let me acknowledge you for wanting to make the world a better place. As I do this, I also acknowledge myself for these accomplishments.

Please hear this message, receive it, and from that place, I invite you (and me) to come out of our hiding places, just one step at a time, knowing that we can retreat there again if we so choose, or we can allow ourselves to be seen in all our fullness and all of our beauty, feeling so calm and content as we do. For when you stand tall and strong and present with the power of who you truly be, then you can invite others to do the same and you can allow any of the dross from other people that may be projected at you to fall away, bearing in mind that it may take some practice to perfect this skill and there may be some hiccups, but they are all part of the practice, and in time, little by little, they will lessen as the pace picks up to let the momentum and flow lead the way.

Chapter 12

CONNECTION

One of our basic needs as humans is connection. And I feel this has been frayed and even fractured to a degree that it has played a big part in the dis-cord, dis-harmony, dis-connection, and dis-ease to varying degrees that we see as individuals and collectively. I believe that a basic desire and even requirement of being human is connection.

That is connection, not just to some form of community or family unit, but connection to our true expanded self. In our body's quest to continually self-heal, it is always guiding us towards that space. And as part of our journey to reconnect to our God self, we will be drawn towards others who can help, which is sometimes perceived as a form of a hindrance; to move towards that place.

In our world today, it is not uncommon to see the breakdown or breakup of family units. Our family unit is where our foundation has been laid. If that does break down and crumble, from scenarios where "dross" has built up and come out as arguments, disagreements then scaled to a level of abuse, physically, mentally, emotionally and even financially, to a point of seemingly no return, then a sense of isolation can be felt, which can lead to further ailments and deep dis-connect.

Even when family units are intact, there can still be a yearning, sometimes even a craving for even more authentic connection.

In a world where there is much focus on instant gratification in the form of fast foods, alcoholic drinks, fake compliments, winning at all costs, short-lived excitement, money, and even sleazy sexual encounters, where do we find true and genuine connection?

Could it be the connection between our small human self to our expanded God self, that could really be the key to sustain and satisfy us in the long term? For that to be strong and lasting, we must work towards becoming energetically aligned to the essence of who we truly be in our greatest sense.

As I write this chapter, I live it. Connection as a theme in my life is challenged. I feel a resistance to connection in my world. I interact in groups, yet I don't feel the connection that I deeply crave. I skirt around the edges. I interject occasionally, then I pull back. Why? I don't even know. It's just what I do. Is it the dross around not fitting in playing out again? I want to connect. I want to be truly part of something, but not really. I know that to fit in somewhere, to really take my place/space at the table, I have to truly own my space.

And that is where my resistance lies. And that brings me to a blank. It's like a dead spot, an evil spot, where I do not live, a spot where I just play the game, dross and all. I know it is there, yet I feel stuck in it, wanting, yet not wanting to shake it off and find my niche, my place in this moment. I want to connect in this one large group or another, yet I don't really want to be seen, and what's more, some of the other members annoy me as they unpack their dross. I care, yet I don't? I am in and I am out, then I settle down, sitting on the fence once again.

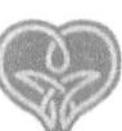

The fence is hard, but it's okay. I can do it. I am used to it really. It is quite comfortable for a bit, then the discomfort sets in and I dip my foot in the water, but it's cold, it's really cold; it's so cold that my breath catches. I gasp for breath. Then I pull it out of that cold water, all the way out, and swing myself all the way around to the other side of the fence, where it is safe, warm, and familiar and my breath flows easily in and out.

I wallow in my dross here. My mind chatter is loud, so loud and so warm that I sink into it. It becomes me and I become it. We embrace like old friends having a reunion and we walk along together and I am alone once again, splashing and swimming in my old patterns of disconnect.

We are all looking for a place where we can be accepted as who we are at this point in time, "warts and all," a genuine community, a transient community, a community that has common threads—a community that is not run by the dross of a few, but by genuine input of all its members. Lots of us are searching for this. It is a common saying to find your tribe. What if you are your tribe? What if you in moving towards your connection to your true expanded self are actually calling in your tribe? What if your tribe is continually changing according to the placement you are on in your individual journey? What if this is true community, inside out and outside in?

We Are One and We Are Many

I can hear the words of that song and see the faces and voices of the children singing it as I write these words. It is such a powerful message in that we are individuals living in our own unique body, yet we have similarities to those around us; our fellow humans. We have similarities in our bodies, minds, and emo-

tions. Our energetic blueprint is also unique, yet more similar than our physical bodies. If we somehow go deeper and expand even further, we arrive at a place where all is one. In the whole big, Universal space, we are all as one, as if everything and everyone merges together as one. This is the space of Source or God. This is a space where all is known and will be revealed at the appropriate time, even though this space knows no time.

It is in our human world that we have created the concept of time. We place great emphasis on time. We need time to function as we do, yet imagine if everything and everyone was functioning from a place of calm, where time didn't exist. We just had day and night and our body guided us through our various fun-filled activities. This is how animals function in their natural state. They eat when they are hungry, play and run when they can, freely express how they feel, and rest and sleep when they are tired.

Chapter 13

BACK TO BASICS

So let's get right back to basics. Let's connect to our earth, our Mother Earth, the ground that we walk on, the elements that give us life, the sense of calm that we feel when we place our bare feet on the raw earth, as we breathe the fresh air, feel the early morning dew against our skin, and soak up the warmth of the sun. This is always such a wonderful place to return us to our calm—our natural state.

Have a look into the word EARTH and rearrange the letters and witness it form the word HEART. What does our heart stand for? Physically, it is the organ that pumps blood around our body, keeping us alive, but is so much more. The earth provides our food, the air we breathe, the water we drink, and the sun to nourish our body and nurture our soul. Our heart is a symbol of love, of connection, and of emotional nourishment. Have a look into the word emotion. It is often said to stand for "energy in motion."

Earth Connection Exercise

Take a moment right now, if possible (or bookmark this page if not), to go stand directly on the earth or imagine that you are standing with your bare feet on the earth. Let yourself become

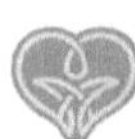

still and present, focus on feeling the fresh air come in through your nose and out the same passage. Feel the sensations in your body as you do this. Is your belly moving, is your chest going up and down, can you feel the air moving inside of your nostrils? Imagine that you are actually breathing with the earth. Then either place your hands above your head or imagine you are doing this and in doing so making direct contact with the sun. Feel the warmth, the strength of the sun soaking into your body, merging with you. Breathe up and down in this manner for three slow breaths. Let your arms relax. Imagine now that your body and surrounding energy field is translucent. Get a feel for that, then sense any dark particles, like droplets of dirt that are floating around here. They represent the dross I have been speaking of. Simply notice them. Then take your awareness down to your feet. Breathe up from your feet and feel the breath come up and out of your head and down around the outside of your body. As the breath comes up so do any of these particles of dross. Let them float down the outside of your body and down to the earth. As they connect with the earth, feel them disappear as they dissolve into the earth. Then the next breath comes up and the process continues. Your breath continues to move up your body, out the top of your head, where it is met by the sun and dispersed outside of your body and into the earth again. The process continues. Let any thoughts that appear be drained away with the dross. After you have finished this process, which can be two minutes or 10 minutes, as long or short as you choose, move your body in a way that feels good for you. You can dance, shake, or move really gently, allowing your intuition to guide you.

If you would like this in an audio format, please email me at healthyhealingwithhelen@gmail.com and I will send it to you.

Soak up the Sunshine

Another exercise I like to do when there is direct sun (not middle of the day): early morning or late afternoon is best. Feet on the earth, if possible, then close your eyes, look at the sun through closed eyes, soak up its healing qualities, including vitamin D, nourishment, and warmth. You can see it as a connection to your expanded self, where you have a direct connection with All That Is and also soak up the wisdom from this space. Be as present as possible and soak it up as you look upwards towards the sun, breathing easily and gently in and out through your nose. Then take a breath in as you open your mouth. As you do this, lift your head and let the sun soak directly into your open mouth. Then drop your head as if you are looking straight ahead, then look down, eyes open, mouth closed. The movement in the jaw here is important too in releasing some of the tension held there. You may cough as you look down. This is just a release of some dross. Continue this exercise for as long as you feel to. When complete, circle your head gently to release any neck tension and do some gentle movement, before moving on to your daily activities.

I want to address some perceptions about the sun and share my truth here. I have utmost reverence for both the sun and the Earth. Yet we have been conditioned to almost fear this sacred light. We are told by the "theys" of the world to cover up, avoid the sun, and apply very heavily chemical-laden lotions and creams to our skin. Reiterating here that our skin is in fact our largest organ and soaks up whatever it comes in contact with, so it is good to be aware of anything you consume through your skin, including sunscreen.

Avoiding the times of day where the sun is at its strongest is always a wise choice, but not always possible, so wearing protective clothing during those times to screen out sun is best and it is also important to choose wisely when using

sunscreens. Find ones that have as few ingredients as possible and are as close to their natural state as possible. Expose yourself and children to natural early morning and late afternoon sun. Seeing gentle sunshine when you first open your eyes rather than artificial light helps the body wake up naturally and sets a healthy precedent for each day.

Do you know that we have receptors in our body that turn on when we go in the sun and tone down the negative effects of excess sun? They are activated by receptors in the eyes. Do you know that wearing sunglasses actually blocks them? Remember that our body will continually do whatever it can to return to its natural state of balance and harmony. The more we can do to assist in this process the better.

Have you ever heard advertising that tells us we have a high chance of getting skin cancer from too much sun? What do you think that advertising campaigns like this one create? Remember the more you hear something, the more likely you are to buy it as real and true and create it in your life.

Everybody is unique. We are born with our own unique blueprint and our own unique body. What is good for one body may not be good for another. That is why it is so important to be present, clear your dross, and follow your awareness of what is best for you at any given point in time.

Your body is your temple, your vehicle to travel through this adventure called life, with as much ease and joy as possible. Connect with it, be present with it, nurture and care for it lovingly, listen to the messages that are for you and you alone. Practise being in a state of calm combined with some common sense, so that you can manoeuvre your way through any turbulence that you encounter with as much serenity as possible.

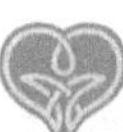

Chapter 14

DOES COMMON SENSE PREVAIL?

The dictionary meaning of common sense is the ability to think and behave in a reasonable way and make sensible decisions. I believe that this is something that keeps us in balance; that is, a state of equilibrium. I also perceive balance as conducive to common sense and in essence, keeping us calm, as individuals and within our world.

We can look at common sense within the concept of receiving information, as in don't believe everything you see or hear. Information is fed through a spectrum of sources, from books to TV or live speaking forums, even music concerts. It can be around something as simple as what to feed ourselves and our children to what part we can play in healing our world. Or are they one and the same?

There are so many ideas and concepts as to what is going on in our world at this time, ranging from high-level corruption, alien invasion, to the Earth rebelling and restructuring. There is much judgement, blame, cruelty, crime, and fighting creating disharmony and chaos, whether it be in the distance or in our neighbourhood. There are extremes of this and there are also extremes on the other side of the coin.

There are so many genuine, caring people speaking out on what is happening, putting forward ideas and concepts on creating real change towards a calmer and healthier world. There are individuals helping each other out in times of crisis. There are some wonderful people caring for animals in need. There are people working behind the scenes on worldwide issues, such as cleaner energy, pure drinking water, healthy healing methods, and more.

And there are individuals like you and me that are focused and committed to creating a happier, healthier, more holistic and balanced life for ourselves and future generations. Whatever we focus on is what we move towards; that is, in what we say, what we think, and how we act. I knew a lady who was continually focused on someone breaking into her car, continually referencing cases where that had happened and talking about it to whoever would listen, and guess what happened? Her car was broken into. I also know someone who has never locked a door in her life, feels safe and happy, and has never experienced any form of break-ins. These are two extremes, then when we add some "common sense" into this scenario, maybe we would keep on locking our doors when required, at the same time as focusing on safety and calm.

Common sense might also say, in general, be aware of what is going on in your neighbourhood and beyond, help out if you are directly called to as guided by your awareness. Be aware that crime is happening, yet don't continually focus on it. In conversation, share stories that are positive and uplifting, instead of focusing and speaking and even judging on what it is you don't like. I very rarely watch "mainstream news," yet always find out whatever I need to, to keep up to date on happenings. Keep your focus on yourself and what you can do

to stay calm and concentrate on what you would like to create in your life and the world at large. Stay in your lane.

There are always opposing points of view as there are two sides of a coin. What if we could BE the coin; that is be in a space of neutrality? See, hear, perceive what is happening from a state of calm, presence and heightened awareness and make choices from that place?

I have most likely introduced you to some new concepts in this book and I suggest using common sense in how to move forward. Keep reading, keep researching, and keep increasing your knowledge and awareness on how you live every day of your life, every footprint you make.

Keep everything in perspective. Use common sense in conjunction with your heightened awareness in making those major decisions, such as moving house, as well as the simple everyday ones, such as what to have for breakfast.

Be aware that there are sources which are incoherently manipulating us in a negative manner in creating more chaos in the form of fear, which can create dis-ease and dis-harmony within our mind and bodies. When we are full of dross and functioning from that space, it is easy to be led along this route.

Explore concepts, techniques, and activities conducive to clearing your dross with an open mind. I have seen people hearing of a new concept or trends and going to extremes, sometimes to their detriment. I am referring to this specifically with healing modalities, nutrition ideas, and even medical treatments. Every interaction you have is based on someone's point of view. Always keep that in mind, notice what feels right for you, do your own research, and explore all other points of

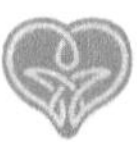

view on any given subject, especially those ones that take a little more investigating to access.

Be aware that things are not always as they appear to be. Sometimes people will appear to be calm and relaxed, yet they have really dropped into a sense of "shut down" in that they have suppressed traumatic or unpleasant situations in their lives and pushed the related dross down really deeply. If this happens, it will often surface as dis-ease, maybe a burst of "out of character" anger or activity at random times.

Chaos can also sometimes be taken out of context. A group of teenagers laughing and partying can appear as chaos. It is sometimes just old-fashioned fun, yet at other times, it can be absolute chaos. Be careful not to confuse chaos with just plain messy. Sometimes messy is a prerequisite to a new era of calm. Look how messy it gets just before you move house. And how calm and relaxed it is once you are unpacked and settled. The studio of an artist is often very messy as they create another masterpiece.

Having a furry four-legged addition to your household can be very messy and even chaotic, especially when they first join your family. What was once your favourite cushion can turn into "snow" around your yard. Your manicured lawn or gardens could become a favourite place to dig. Little accidents can appear in places you don't expect. And all this interspersed with periods of calm and cuteness overload. As time goes on and the love and connection expand, an extra sense of calm can spread throughout your life.

Chapter 15

FOR THE LOVE OF A DOG

I feel that I need to address "man's best friend" at this point. If you reverse the letters in the word DOG, it spells GOD. I see all animals as sentient beings. They are here on Earth to play their individual role and live out their lives with as much calm and contentment as possible. Animals complement us in a variety of ways, as do plants. Imagine if there was a mutual respect and caring for plants, animals, and humans and we lived in harmony on the Earth. Still room for overall improvement here, but there are some amazing people playing a brilliant role in creating that in their areas of expertise.

So back to dogs, who live in close connection to humans. I feel that having a dog or close relationship with any animal can be such a contribution to creating calm in one's life and even helping in clearing our dross, whether it be as a trigger for something for us to look at and clear or such a deep love and energetic connection.

I didn't grow up around dogs, although my grandfather always had one. We did not have a dog as a pet in our family, as my mother didn't hold a high opinion of them. She thought that dogs were dirty, a nuisance, a waste of money, spread germs, and generally would be too much trouble, all of which I subconsciously took

on, and as a result, my children never had a dog either as they grew up, even though there were some requests.

It wasn't until I was 50 and well on a journey of clearing my dross and subconscious patterning that I got my first dog. My older son and daughter had left home by this time and adopted a dog of their own and I immediately became a "Puppy Grandma" and found out that this was a role I really enjoyed.

My youngest daughter was still living at home and had always wanted a dog so, without hesitation, we adopted one. His name was Leo and he was a Staffy. Little did I know that having him would add a whole new dimension to my life. It was so liberating to see that none of the previous points of view that I had about dogs were mine at all. This is such a classic example of how clearing your dross works, in you becoming more of yourself and discovering the real you.

The first step in inviting Leo into our home was learning the physical aspects of feeding, walking, training, and scooping poop, then working with behaviour and learning how to read his energy and body language. Little did I know that scooping the poop was actually the easy part.

Being a puppy parent is a continual journey with many ups and downs, but the depth of love and connection that I had for this dog was off the charts. And not just him, but dogs in general. I had actually always liked them, yet now I became obsessed with these animals, continually learning what I could about them and deriving so much joy from seeing dogs being cared for, running and playing on the beach, and generally having fun. Leo has now passed, yet as I write this, I look at his picture smiling at me and remember him fondly.

After Leo, I couldn't imagine myself without a dog, so not long after his passing, Atlas came into our family. He has brought with

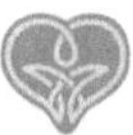

him another level of trials and tribulations. My journey with him has been filled with many tears, as well as many tender moments, as my learning not just about him but about myself continues.

I remember one of the best pieces of advice I received when Atlas first came to live with us as a puppy was to always remember that he is a dog, not a little person. And I think that is where a lot of kind, caring people have problems with their animals in that they cross that line and treat them like children. They do have similarities in they require a high level of care, yet we need to continually remind ourselves of the obvious differences and find that very fine line to help us become in sync with them to gift and receive in more ways than one.

Having a dog can be such a source of mutual connection on all planes from physical to energetic. There will be moments of calm and moments of chaos. You will be forced to learn more about energy as this is how they communicate. They can bring that sense of connection that you may be longing for and they will deepen your sense of love for them and open an opportunity for you to love yourself more deeply than you previously had, if you can see yourself through their eyes.

Self-love is something that is often referred to in spiritual teachings. I believe that the more of our dross or negative conditioning that we clear, the more this will automatically happen. So much of our dross revolves around not being good enough, smart enough, and being riddled with so much fear at the concept of sharing what we truly think, feel, and desire. As it clears and releases, you will begin to know yourself more fully and naturally move towards being one with your expanded or GOD self, which I believe in many cases is how your dog sees you. We see them as a DOG and I wonder if they see us as GOD?

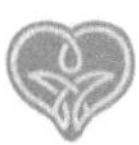

Chapter 16

CONTROL VERSUS FREEDOM

Animals live with a sense of freedom just doing their thing, whether that be relaxing or running or playing, all the while communicating with their energetic self, yet as humans our life is more controlled. I wonder if we could find a balance in letting go of an element of control to allow for a calm sense of freedom and in that, less chaos.

If I think of the energy of control, it seems quite set and rigid, yet if we overlay it with a sense of calm, it somehow merges into freedom. The energy becomes much more flowing and expansive. Then, if that freedom gets out of control, we can have chaos. Seems like a vicious cycle, with what could be seen as a very fine line between these energies.

The dictionary meaning of control is "the power to influence or direct people's behaviour or the course of events." Control in our lives today can be perceived as a necessary evil. It is a force which can be used as simple guidance with freedom still in place or it can be a force of great destructive power and chaos.

As children, we do require some form of control to guide us into respectable adult members of society. If this control comes

in the form of simple loving guidance from teachers, parents, and carers who can be present and clear, then it would allow each individual to find their own source of individual power and creativity to grow into a happy, healthy, self-respecting adult.

When control is coming from someone in a chaotic state full of dross, then it can be a destructive force. You can see this in large organisations, that are totally focused on power and greed, exerting control over people as they fall prey to their manipulation techniques. Control often works in subtle and sneaky ways and is not always detected with our five senses, and can create large-scale chaos or individual chaos.

As an individual, as we clear our dross, heighten our awareness, and improve our connection to our expanded God self, we can see the places where this is happening. When enough people can see this, and shine their light upon it, it will have nowhere to hide and as it is exposed, even more people will be able to see it in its early phases, giving it a chance to course correct and meander its way towards freedom.

Freedom, "the power or right to act, speak or think as one chooses," compared to control, which means "the power to influence or direct people's behaviour or the course of events."

Can you see a strong variant from the formal meaning of control? Can you see the correlation between these two words? Imagine if they danced together, as in our behaviour was directed in a calm, loving, clear manner.

Helen Melrose

As you read this particular chapter, I invite you to take some slow breaths and allow the energetic transmission beneath these words to soak and merge within your energy field.

Let me end this chapter with a poem that I wrote in 1998:

FROM FEAR TO FREEDOM

We must Feel Fragile and Frail to appreciate our Fullness

We must Feel the Finality of an experience to allow it to Finish

We must Finish an experience to allow the Future to come
to Fruition

We must Finally see the Futility of our eFForts and let them go

We must experience the Finiteness to enable us to move
towards the inFinity of ourselves

We must Feel an aFFinity with members of our Family

We must become Fond of ourselves and Follow our dreams

We must use our Failures to Fathom our Future

We must Fumble and Falter towards Freedom

We must have Fun in the light Fantastic

We must Face our Fears to Frame our Future

LET'S MAKE OUR FUTURE FREE FROM FEAR AND
FULL OF FREEDOM

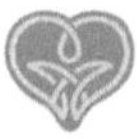

Chapter 17

FROM GRANDMA WITH LOVE

I received my greatest birthday gift as I turned 54, with the birth of my first granddaughter, born from my eldest daughter. I took on the title of Grandma with such pride and joy. Today I have four granddaughters and one grandson, born as I do the final edit for this book. I have so much Love for each of these precious children.

Being a grandma is a role that I truly relish and one that brings me much joy. I can still remember the moment that each of them first said the word Grandma in their cute, tiny one-year-old voice. It just melted my heart, as does every Grandma cuddle.

I am very blessed that all of my grandchildren live very close and I get to see them regularly, witness their milestone moments, and watch them grow and develop. It is also such a gift to me to see my children in the role of parents and how well they play this role. Being a grandma as well as being a mum is something that I take very seriously as well as light-heartedly in acknowledging the blessing bestowed upon me, in playing it.

My first role in being a "mum" started when I was just a child. In my family, my mother did an amazing job of taking care

of the physical and mental needs of all of us children at the highest possible level and Dad worked two, sometimes three jobs to make sure that financially we had all that we required. Somehow, as the eldest girl, with my parents so busy, I became a second mum to my younger siblings and loved caring and cuddling and playing with them. I just naturally fell into this role and really did enjoy it, and unknowingly at the time was practising for future mothering roles I would play.

We had a pleasant childhood, a comfortable home, and lots of neighbourhood friends to play with and every toy and yummy thing a child could want. However, my teenage years gave me plenty of dross to clear and lots of opportunities to learn. Of course, at that time, I couldn't see them and fell into a pattern of resisting, reacting, and continually blaming something or someone, usually my mother, which ultimately only hurt me. Now I can see that time in my life in a different light and know that those experiences have contributed to helping me become a better parent and grandparent.

I digress here and take a trip down memory lane to include an excerpt from a day in my life as a young mother. The year was 1996 and my key role was of a full-time mother.

Mum the Magician

"I believe that mothering is the most underrated, underpaid, yet most important and rewarding job there is. Unless you've been there yourself, I don't believe you realise how busy and stressful that parenting can be. I have to admit that, before I had children of my own, I thought that mothers who stayed home spent their days pegging out a bit of washing, maybe pushing the kids on the swings, reading a story or two and maybe coffee with friends, while the children played happily together. How easy could it be?

However, four children later, I now realise that there is so much more involved—not just physically, but mentally and emotionally as well. And to illustrate this, I am going to share a day in my life as Mum. This day started at 5 a.m. with the sound of my real live alarm clock. I tried to ignore it after a sleepless night, but couldn't, so got up and changed a nappy and fed my baby girl and thought I would put her in bed with me and she would go back to sleep and I could get a bit more shut-eye, but within minutes the entire contents of my bedside table had landed on the floor. I ducked just in time to miss the corner of a book in my eye and took this as the cue to get up.

I locked baby gates, put a dead cockroach and open pencil case out of reach and started piling the first load of washing in the machine. She was happy to toddle around for a bit, while I started making lunches— three lunchboxes and one esky to fill, all with home-cooked, healthy food, of course. One by one the rest of the family woke up and proceeded to devour a pot of rolled oats I was looking forward to. I finally filled all the lunchboxes, when my older son informed me that he didn't need any lunch today. 'Remember, Mum,' he said. 'I told you last week that we are having an international food day today and I have to take a fruit salad.' I wasn't impressed but somehow managed to put together a fruit salad. Next daughter was happy with her lunch, but where was her sports uniform? Why wasn't it hanging up in her wardrobe, when she needed it? 'I suppose I won't be able to play sport today—because of you,' she said in her 'little miss' voice. I gave her 'the look' and she disappeared back into her room only to reappear ten minutes later wearing the missing attire.

The older kids packed up and rode their bikes off to school; I loaded the two little ones into the car along with the bowl of fruit salad, which was left sitting on the bench after they had

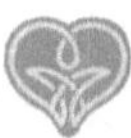

gone, and off we went for kindy drop-off, dropping off the fruit salad at school on the way. I finally left the kindergarten with one child crying because he didn't want to stay and the other crying because she didn't want to leave.

But eventually we did leave and headed home. Baby asleep and I proceed to peg out washing till the line was full and the peg basket empty. Next, I cleaned the kitchen and tidied up enough that I could walk around the house without feeling like I was completing an obstacle course or sticking and crunching on who knows what. I was just about to sit down with that much-anticipated cup of coffee when baby was awake and demanding attention again. Pretty soon, we were in the car and off to the shops. I kept trying to convince myself how easy it was shopping with one little girl, not yet talking, compared to two, three, or even four children, all full of wants.

When my trolley was full and my purse empty, I came home, unpacked the groceries, brought in washing, did kindy pick-up, then prepared for this afternoon's activities, which today was netball. At the netball courts, I parted with a little bit more money and spent the next hour with one eye on the court and the other on the younger children, one fighting over sitting on the same chair as another little boy, and the other taste-testing as many drink bottles as she could lay her hands on. Then just as we were about to leave, she somehow managed to trip with a drink bottle in her hand and cut her lip.

I cleaned it up and comforted her as best I could, then reluctantly put her back in that dreaded car seat along with her three siblings and it was home for the day to prepare dinner, bathing duties, and eventually younger children's bedtime. When they were in bed, there were dishes to do, washing to sort, sequins to sew, homework to help with, then finally bed.

In this job, where there is no formal training, one needs to be creative, organised, versatile, and energetic and to fill the roles of cleaner, cook, chauffeur, nurse, bookkeeper, referee, gardener, and even magician, sometimes at only a minute's notice.

The pay is nil and the hours are long, but as challenging as it may appear, I believe that our future and that of future generations depends on how well it is performed, and the rewards surpass the currency of money and are delivered in experiencing the role of mother from different angles and aspects as we move through life."

And the ultimate gift for me was to be elevated into the role of Grandma.

Parenting is such a huge learning curve and as you wind your way through it, you are almost certain to stumble and fall. But it is in the getting back up, dusting off some of the dross and the judgement of where it came from, then moving forward, that once again more dross is cleared. Or you can climb onto that element of rightness and in it gather some more dross, maybe even an extra load as you add some from your "rightness aligners."

Playing the grandma role is like the icing on the cake. It's as if you have graduated from that real hands-on parenting role into a role where you can enjoy the moments with the children, relish in their beauty and playfulness, know the importance of being present with them, and now have the time to do just that. There is something so special for a child and grandparent to spend time together and be present with each other.

As Grandma, I love squishing home-made Play-Doh through my fingers, acting out in play roles, especially those ones where

they say, "You be the sister and I'll be the mum." I also love snuggling up with a story book at sleep time, as well as cheering them on as they perform in their chosen activities. Each aspect is a two-way gift in itself. And has an extra bonus as their mum and dad have some time with each other.

Another benefit of being a grandma is seeing your children as parents and watching their reaction as their children act out, just as they did at their age. This has certainly given me a few laughs, a few cringes, and some proud Mumma moments.

And let me iterate here that the "Grandma" role can be played by anyone. Imagine if we somehow found a way to connect young children in day care while Mum and Dad are at work to having some time with possibly elderly residents of a nursing home. This could be an opening for some magic to happen in more ways than one.

The essence of my message here is that our children are our future. And the experiences that they have on all levels are so important. They are the foundation upon which our future is laid. Never underestimate the power of the transference of your wisdom and life's experiences to the next generation and beyond. What if we could deliver the energy of calm, serenity, and honouring of ourselves into this generation, so that they can weather the storms that are occurring and will continue, until the majority of us have cleared enough of the dross to glide through that gap in the fence into a future we are all destined to enjoy.

Chapter 18

TIPS FOR CREATING MORE CALM

I refer a lot about clearing the dross to move towards a calmer, healthier place in life and am referring to this from an energetic perspective, as that is where the clearing happens, then filters through into your everyday life, sometimes in ways that have no logical sense, such as when I noticed that my concept around what I thought about dogs had changed. This was not something I consciously set out to change, yet it opened up my life to an extra level of joy and deep learning by adding another whole dimension to it.

In other instances, I have set out to change or heal a certain aspect of my personality or a health issue that is no longer serving me and it has shifted over time. One example was when I had a frozen shoulder, that I was told would need surgery. I was guided to a series of natural therapy treatments as well as visualisation, movement, and healing energy for my physical body and fully healed it without any form of medical intervention.

As I write this book and embody its teachings, once again, more of my dross comes up. I am much more comfortable staying

behind the scenes and living in my own bubble. My perceived failed attempts at exposing myself in my fullness are coming up yet again and my very well-defined patterns of giving up are trying to coax me back into my safe space. My physical body is aching and my mind racing. Over and over, I use whatever techniques I am drawn to; to keep on keeping on clearing all that presents itself as best I can, so that I can return to that space of presence and look forward to what I would like to create for my future and beyond.

Having a healthy physical body and clear mind is conducive to a calm demeanour. Taking responsibility for your state of health and keeping your body and ultimately your life in the most natural state as possible is conducive to creating just that. What if you could be your own doctor? What if you could tune into your unique body's desire to heal itself and move towards a state of good health and wellbeing? What if you could allow yourself to be led to healing methods that are in alignment with what is paramount to creating a greater sense of calm in your physical body as well as your mental, emotional, and spiritual self? Using "preventative" and "alternate" medicine and therapies is not encouraged so much or supported by authorities at this time, yet they have a huge role to play in our journey towards calm.

Taking responsibility for your own health and exploring different modalities and treatments that are in alignment with the individual that you are, as well as clearing your dross, which is what I did in healing my shoulder, is a journey in itself. It is not always an easy or straightforward path as our societal conditioning sends us straight into treatments, which often jump immediately to using toxic chemical substances and surgical procedures. What if we could also know when traditional medical treatment and possibly surgical procedures

are required and be of such gratitude that this is possible? What if all treatments could complement each other, with an element of mutual respect and gratitude?

What if assessing food, nutrition, and exercise was the first "port of call" to any healing journey? What if this was started at an early age? I know that plenty of people do this, as I was just at my local organic farmers market and it was buzzing. Yet I know that big supermarkets and pharmacies are also busy and many trolleys are chock-full of processed food. Everything that is presented for sale is guided by you and I as the consumer and changes along with our preferences.

What if we started to be aware of what processed foods we consumed and gradually reduced them, as we looked for natural alternatives and made some conscious steps towards more healthy food choices? A potful of fresh basil, parsley, or mint grown on your balcony and added to a meal will give you more goodness than any processed foods by a mile. Garlic is a natural antibiotic and contributes to healing dis-ease or physical imbalance as can many common herbs and even plants we refer to as weeds, as I mentioned earlier. Growing your own herbs and vegetables is a very satisfying activity on all levels.

Preparing and cooking plant-based meals is a real eye-opener as to how much scope and real yumminess there is here. This is something that I have learnt from scratch and an activity I really enjoy, yet I know is not everybody's "cup of tea." There are, however, plenty of local people preparing and cooking fresh, healthy meals. I believe it is always good to support small businesses in your area. I personally still buy some processed foods, but over time have minimised them greatly. Reading labels when shopping is a good habit to incorporate. The smaller the list of ingredients, the better.

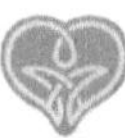

As I mentioned earlier, I brought up my children from a natural health perspective as best I could, learning along the way. I remember one of the things I didn't agree with was amalgam fillings in teeth and was ridiculed at that time by dentists and health providers, yet I stood my ground. Now, just 30 years later, the problems with this toxic substance have been exposed and it is no longer used.

The more of us that wake up to knowing what does and does not contribute to a greater sense of good health across all areas of society and stand up for our truths, the more things will change. I know that at this point in time, it looks like things are getting worse, but I also know that more people are clearing their dross and in turn becoming more aware and waking up to what really works across all levels of the playing field and what does not.

Having a happy, healthy mouth and teeth is something that is conducive to good health throughout our whole body. The health of our teeth affects the overall health of our body in a multitude of ways. In some healing modalities, certain teeth relate to certain areas of the body. Knowing this can help when healing imbalances within our body. Be aware that how you breathe can affect your teeth and jaw alignment. There is an interesting book by James Nestor titled *Breath: The New Science of a Lost Art* that addresses this concept in detail.

My youngest daughter had extremely crowded teeth when she was young and was advised to have teeth removed and orthodontic treatment. I looked into other alternatives, hoping to avoid teeth extraction, and found a modality called orthotropics. It works in addressing cranial and jaw alignment and correcting the breathing. We embarked on treatment for both her and her brother. Neither

of them had any teeth removed and now almost 20 years later, both have a strong, healthy jaw, and straight, well-aligned teeth.

Using a natural toothpaste and not cleaning teeth directly after a meal is a good practice. This is because the mouth is quite acid after eating and needs to be alkaline for best cleaning results. Rinsing with a combination of salt and good quality bi-carb soda can help to alkalise the mouth before brushing if required. Oil pulling, which is swishing the mouth with coconut or olive oil for five to 15 minutes, then discarding it, can help to keep the mouth clean as it pulls toxins from the mouth. Adding good-quality clove and cinnamon essential oils to this mix is an option. This is just a snippet of information on oral health. I suggest reading and researching this area for more information. One book I found helpful here is *Holistic Dental Care* by Nadine Artemis.

Let me just touch on essential oils here as they can be such a potent healing tool. My favourite would have to be lavender oil. It is very calming and soothing for nerves as well as having antiseptic qualities. Enjoying a lavender bath allows this oil to soak into all those cracks and crevices in our body that simply get washed over in a shower. Essential oils can be used in a wide range of healing instances, ranging from insect bites to easing the symptoms of commons colds and tummy upset. Some oils such as peppermint are uplifting while others have a calming effect. There is much information on this topic. I hope you will read further and implement what works for you and your family. One of my old favourites on this topic is *The Enchanting Art of Aromatherapy* by Savatore Battaglia.

Did you know that we hold more tension in the jaw than any other area of our body? Being aware of this and doing what

you can to release tight jaw muscles is always helpful and in particular may even free up and release tension in the pelvic area. A relaxed jaw has a multitude of health benefits. Just being aware of when you clench your jaw and even hold your breath is helpful, so that you can focus on consciously relaxing and stretching this section of your body.

As I continually say in my classes, breathing and moving release tension from the body, while holding the breath as you move can create tension and ultimately discomfort. Remembering to stop and breathe, especially when in a stressful situation, is so calming in itself. Take a moment now and notice your breath. Is it slow and deep or shallow or quick?

One easy breathing technique I would like to share is: breathe in through your nose slowly as you count to three (or more), feel your belly gently rise as you do this, then pause and let the breath out slowly again as you count to four or five.(the key is to make the out breathe longer than the in breath). Try it and see how relaxed you feel.

Something else to be really aware of in a practical sense is keeping the use of technology in balance. Again, it has its place and is so helpful in many ways, but is it overused? What if social media, TV, and even movies were used as an adage to spending time in nature, physical contact with friends, and healthy exercise activities?

This is really important with children as they are learning and growing at a rate much faster than adults. As children, their foundations for adulthood are being laid. Anyone who has influence in their lives has the responsibility, or I would even go as far as to say privilege, to influence them in a way that is positive or negative.

This includes providers of media and anything that children respond to. What if TV could have a positive effect and increase learning in ways that will benefit them as they grow? As a caregiver, it is our role to be aware of what our children are watching and in effect, absorbing through TV and other media outlets. TV screens have grown to exorbitant sizes, to the point where the characters are sometimes as big as or bigger than us, and in our "zombie" state we can go into when watching something, it can be hard to distinguish what is real and what is not. This can be conducive or detrimental in creating more overall calm.

Again, everything comes down to clearing our dross and being guided more from our expanded God self and continuing to question. Question what does not "feel right" and also use the humble question as a healing tool. As in when you are unsure or wobbly about an issue or decision you have to make, then turn it into a question and send it out to the Universe without any expectations, then notice any signs or signals that are presented to you.

Be aware that this is a journey to a destination that is constantly changing, with ups and downs and twists and turns. To ride those waves, be as gentle as possible on yourself and do whatever you can to continually bring yourself back towards that state of calm and of presence.

Over the years, I have used many different and varied healing modalities to move through some times of turbulence. While I find myself in more of an overall space of calm, my journey and clearing continues as I wind my way through whatever life presents to me in any moment. I have studied and practised such modalities as nutrition, bodywork, reflexology, NLP, kinesiology, massage, EFT

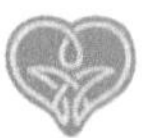

tapping, aromatherapy, jaw reset, access bars, spiritual healing, counselling, life coaching, meditation, numerology, homeopathy, yoga teaching, and peiec energy healing in working towards clearing my own dross.

I encourage everyone to devote some time in their day to self-healing or relaxation practices, using whatever techniques or tools work for you. I have a morning routine, where I spend some time being still, present, breathing gently, and acknowledging myself for doing my best at whatever point I am at in my life as well as reminding myself and sending gratitude for all that I have in my life. Then I focus on activities conducive to clearing some dross and heightening my connection to my expanded self.

Some days I will do a short relaxation or meditation exercise, some form of physical movement as well as an energetic clearing. On other days, I am up early taking my dog for a walk, doing whatever job is required, or lying in bed with a cup of tea and a good book. Today I started my day with a warm lemon water, then out for a walk on the beach and swim in the salt water with my partner and dog.

It is important to find a routine that fits naturally into your lifestyle and allows for flexibility when required. I use my Energetic Reset exercises and Morphogenie Healing as I am guided. A spiritual practice is not something that is forced or creates extra stress. It is uniquely yours and honouring of you as a spiritual being as well as in your physical reality. Going for a bushwalk and soaking up the energy of the majestic trees you pass can be a spiritual practice. How you live your life is a spiritual practice in itself.

I love to connect with nature and find solace there. When walking in the bush or on the beach, if I have something

challenging happening in my life, I will allow my thoughts to go rampant for a certain amount of time, then I will stop and maybe go the other direction if I am on the beach or turn a corner if I am on a bush walk. At that point, I focus on my breath, clear my mind, and bring myself into a space of presence as best I can. Sometimes I will hum or count or even speak some "gibberish" to keep those thoughts at bay.

Journalling is also something that I find quite cathartic and can assist in moving from a state of chaos towards more calm. Sometimes I will write like crazy, then burn the paper and let go of some dross in that manner. Other times I will write to find some consistency and clarity in whatever may be troubling me. Other times I will journal my reasons to have gratitude to really reiterate the importance of all that I have in my life.

Focusing on gratitude is a powerful exercise in itself. Some people like to keep a gratitude journal and use it every day. Having reminders around your main living area can be a good tool to help come back to a calm space of gratitude when the chaos gets overwhelming. There used to be, and still is, to a certain extent, a focus on positive thinking. While I don't believe that you can "think" yourself to a space of calm, I do feel that keeping your language as well as thoughts in a positive manner can certainly contribute, in the context of what you focus on expands.

Today I am about to finish off a 24-hour fast. I was feeling a bit sluggish and generally off, so was guided to do this to create some healing in my physical body. I am about to make a smoothie using celery, beetroot, garlic, ginger, as well as some greens from my garden to nourish my body to break the fast and will slowly introduce fresh fruit and vegetables into my diet today.

In my life, I am aware of what I eat and ingest in all areas, without being obsessed, as well as doing plenty of movement activities. I prioritise and incorporate spiritual practices I feel guided to into my life, as well as activities that are fun and bring me joy. I like to do this outside where possible so I have a direct connection to the earth. I appreciate all that our natural world has to offer and commune in places that have that connection.

CONCLUSION

Let me acknowledge you for reading this far and allowing the energetic component of these words to permeate into your energetic space. I am hoping that you will feel a greater sense of presence and of calm in this moment, as well as an inkling or even a sense of enthusiasm to take some of the ideas from this book and incorporate them into your life. I hope that you will have more awareness of the importance of clearing your dross and connecting more with your expanded energetic self and perceiving your life and making choices from that vantage point.

I have read so many books and received so much healing and pleasure and taken on board and instigated teachings from many of them. I have participated in a variety of courses and programs, healing circles, and women's retreats in person and now, at this time mostly online, over many years. I have used some of them for varying amounts of time and others, I have had the learning that this is not for me and left it "on the table," so to speak. I have gathered the knowledge I present in this book from these teachings and implementing them into my life's experiences.

My path has wound around lots of different directions and sometimes seemed to have looped in circles. I see the world from a different perspective than the vast majority of people and have resisted and judged and fought and complained about a lot of what is going on. Yet I know that I am here at this time in our evolution, as are you, to contribute to making our world

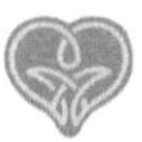

a better place, where the energy of calm increases and infuses into places and spaces currently filled with chaos and dross.

Imagine you have such a strong sense of calm that you can truly honour the sovereignty of yourself on all levels. You are clear on your role in this journey we call life. You notice the happenings around you and know when to take action and when to send some loving thoughts. You hear the opinions of others, yet they don't affect you in a negative manner, allowing you to stay in your lane and on your unique path with confidence and ease. Imagine all areas of your life are flowing and in balance. Get a sense of this, for this is what you tap into when you go through that gap in the fence.

My focus for myself and my family is on the future. I acknowledge the past, but do not dwell on it or try to dissect it. I look forward to a future for all of us, where a sense of calm prevails, as we create all of our desires with a sense of ease, fun, and mutual respect for all life.

In conclusion I will ask of you to:

Be the best person you possibly can, under the circumstances you presently find yourself.

Accept where you and those around you are at, whether it be chaos or calm or somewhere in between.

Be kind and loving to yourself first, then let those qualities move outwards to wherever you are guided.

Always extend your comfort zone, but never push into any pain.

See your life as a dance, as in taking steps in one direction, then another, moving easily and gracefully.

Give yourself permission to rest and integrate when required.

Step out of your bubble to expose your unique beauty and brilliance.

Ask for and accept help when required, from whatever source you may be led.

Offer help when it is asked for.

Continually express gratitude for the simple things.

Treat others how you would like to be treated.

Honour and nurture your physical body.

Let your voice be heard.

Hear the voices of those around you.

Acknowledge where others are at in their journey and have compassion.

Walk away when you need to and engage when guided.

Have as much fun as possible in whatever you choose to do.

Sing, dance, laugh, move, play.

Keep learning and discerning.

Continually strive for more and more connection to your true expanded self that is directly connected to God/Source/ Universe/All That Is.

Stay true to your inner most truth.

Know that you matter and have an integral part to play in creating more calm in your life and beyond.

Much Love and Blessings
Helen

SUMMARY OF AWARENESS REMINDERS FOR PRACTICAL IDEAS TOWARDS CREATING MORE CALM

Awareness as a Reminder:

- Continually reminder yourself to use your own awareness in whatever you do
- Stay in your lane as you listen to the points of views and teachings of others
- Take on only what resonates with you
- Stand tall and strong in your point of view without moving into and getting stuck in rightness
- Be flexible enough to see things from different angles

Clearing Energetic Dross:

- Understand the concept and importance of clearing energetic dross
- Explore ways to shift perspectives and open up to new dimensions of joy and learning
- Use the humble question as a powerful tool to allow for new opportunities and ideas to manifest as well as continually questioning what doesn't feel right for you and your body
- Embrace the journey of constant change, acknowledging ups and downs, and moving with them with as much ease and grace as possible

Holistic Health Approach:

- Take responsibility for your health and explore natural self-healing methods
- Use natural healing methods such as poultices, cold compresses

- Garlic and onion in home healing can work wonders
- Use good-quality essential oils to enhance relaxation, upliftment, and cleansing
- Be open to alternate healing modalities as guided by your awareness
- Use and be grateful for medical treatments when required

Food and Nourishment:

- Be mindful of what you eat and regularly nourish your body with foods that are as close to their natural state as possible
- Be aware of how, when, and why you eat and feed your body with the reverence it deserves
- Consider integrating fasting as a healing tool for the physical body
- Grow some simple herbs and vegetables to use each day

Nutrition and Exercise:

- Assess food, nutrition, and exercise as primary elements in your healing journey
- Gradually reduce processed foods, opting for natural alternatives
- Support local businesses that provide fresh and healthy meal options

Oral Health Awareness:

- Understand the impact of oral health on overall wellbeing
- Opt for toothpaste without harmful substances and practise oil pulling for mouth detoxification
- Clean your teeth when your mouth is alkaline

Conscious Movement Practices

- Practise stretching, moving to release your body consciously in sync with breath
- Be aware of jaw tension and its connection to overall body tension
- Incorporate conscious breathing, especially in stressful situations
- Try a simple breathing technique: inhale slowly for a count, pause, and exhale slowly for a slightly longer count
- Be aware of mouth breathing as this can affect the alignment of the jaw and much more
- Check you are breathing through your nose

Journalling and Gratitude:

- Journalling can be cathartic; burn paper to let go of dross or write for consistency and clarity
- Emphasise gratitude; maintain a gratitude journal or use reminders to shift focus during overwhelming moments

Positive Language and Thinking:

- Be aware of your thoughts and words
- Keep language towards yourself and others positive; focus on what you want to expand
- Understand the power of positive language in contributing to an overall state of calm

Use Technology Wisely:

- Keep technology use in balance; use social media and screens mindfully

- Prioritise spending time in nature, physical contact with friends, and engaging in healthy exercise activities
- Be mindful of the content both you and your children are exposed to on TV and media
- Consider positive effects and learning opportunities that media can provide when used consciously

Morning Routine for Presence:

- Establish a morning routine that includes stillness, breath awareness, and acknowledgment of your efforts
- Focus on activities conducive to clearing dross and heightening the connection to your expanded self
- Find solace in nature; walk on the beach or in the bush to clear the mind and calm the nervous system
- Practise presence by becoming aware of thoughts, then letting them go as you focus on the here and now
- How you live your life is a spiritual practice in itself

Energetic Reset Practices:

- Engage in energetic clearing techniques learned through various modalities
- Choose movement activities and exercises that connect you directly to the earth
- Honour and acknowledge the healing qualities of the earth and the sun and use them wisely

These are but a few reminders towards creating a calmer lifestyle. Keep things in perspective. Do what works for you in any given moment. Continue to be open to new teachings that feel aligned. And most of all, acknowledge and honour your connection to your God self and continue to foster that relationship.

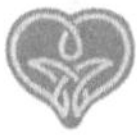

What if there is no right or wrong or good or bad, only learning, growing, moving, shifting, and changing, all in perfect timing?

Extra Support

From my experience and experimentation with different modalities combined with accessing and drawing upon my expanded self, I have prepared a very simple, short online course called "Energetic Reset" that you can use to incorporate a regular spiritual practice into your life as well as gently clearing some dross.

For an extra level of support, I offer individual Morphogenie Healing sessions. Sessions are tailored for your unique requirements, releasing dross energetically to move into a space of more wholeness and calm, in an easy gentle manner.

I also offer in-person yoga/conscious movement classes in my local area, which are a combination of yoga, qi gong, Feldenkrais, Pilates, and breath work with a lovely relaxation at the end.

For further information, please go to my website

www.healthyhealingwithhelen.com

Or follow me on my Facebook page,

Healthy Healing with Helen

Or email me on healthyhealingwithhelen@gmail.com

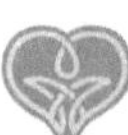

ACKNOWLEDGMENTS

I would like to acknowledge Dave, Davina, and the amazing team from Inspirational Book Writers in bringing this book into physical form. They have all supported and encouraged me to bring an intangible mishmash of ideas and concepts into the tangible form in which you find it in today.

I would like to extend a huge thank you to my four amazing adult children, Matthew, Tahnee, Brenton, and Neroli, each of whom I am immensely proud, for carving out their own unique pathway in such a loving and caring manner, as they journey through life; to their wonderful spouses and beautiful children. As well as a special thank you to my awesome partner Les. I am so blessed to have such a loving and supportive family and give thanks each and every day. I would like to add an extra thank you to Neroli in creating the cover design and photo for this book.

I would like to acknowledge the spiritual healers and teachers who have assisted and guided me in clearing my dross, raising my vibration to bring me closer to my expanded God self. To many kind, caring friends I have interacted with over the years and who continue to support me. To my wonderful yoga community, some of whom have been coming to my classes over many years and to those who will join in future time, I thank and acknowledge you. I would like to thank everyone

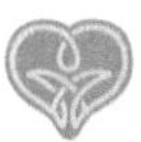

who has allowed me the privilege of facilitating you into a space of calm as the dross creating chaos in your life drips away. And most of all, I would like to acknowledge and thank you, the reader, for reading my words, receiving the energy, living your best life, and contributing to creating a better world for us and for future generations.

Notes

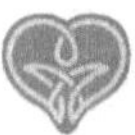

Notes

Notes

Notes

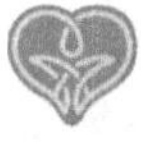

Notes

www.ingramcontent.com/pod-product-compliance
Lightning Source LLC
Chambersburg PA
CBHW051102250726
48656CB00001B/428